<u>Introduction</u>

After struggling with my own weight for the past 25 years, and basically trying many diets in the process of losing it, I decided to simplify what really works and show this in a more visual way, without many words or explanations and without spending money in the process.

I have lost over 30 pounds over the past few years; the last 10 pounds I lost a year ago, and I have kept it all off since then. I feel great and healthy!

This book was created with the sole intention to share with my fellow humans, the way losing weight really worked for me, and that I didn't have to spend any money to lose the weight. The contents of this book are not intended to replace any medical or professional advice.

==========

My deepest appreciation to my wife Daisy, for her support, for allowing me the time and for allowing me to be myself. And to my children: Armando E, Raphael J, Monica A, and Alexander T.; who are truly great young adults.

Find today...

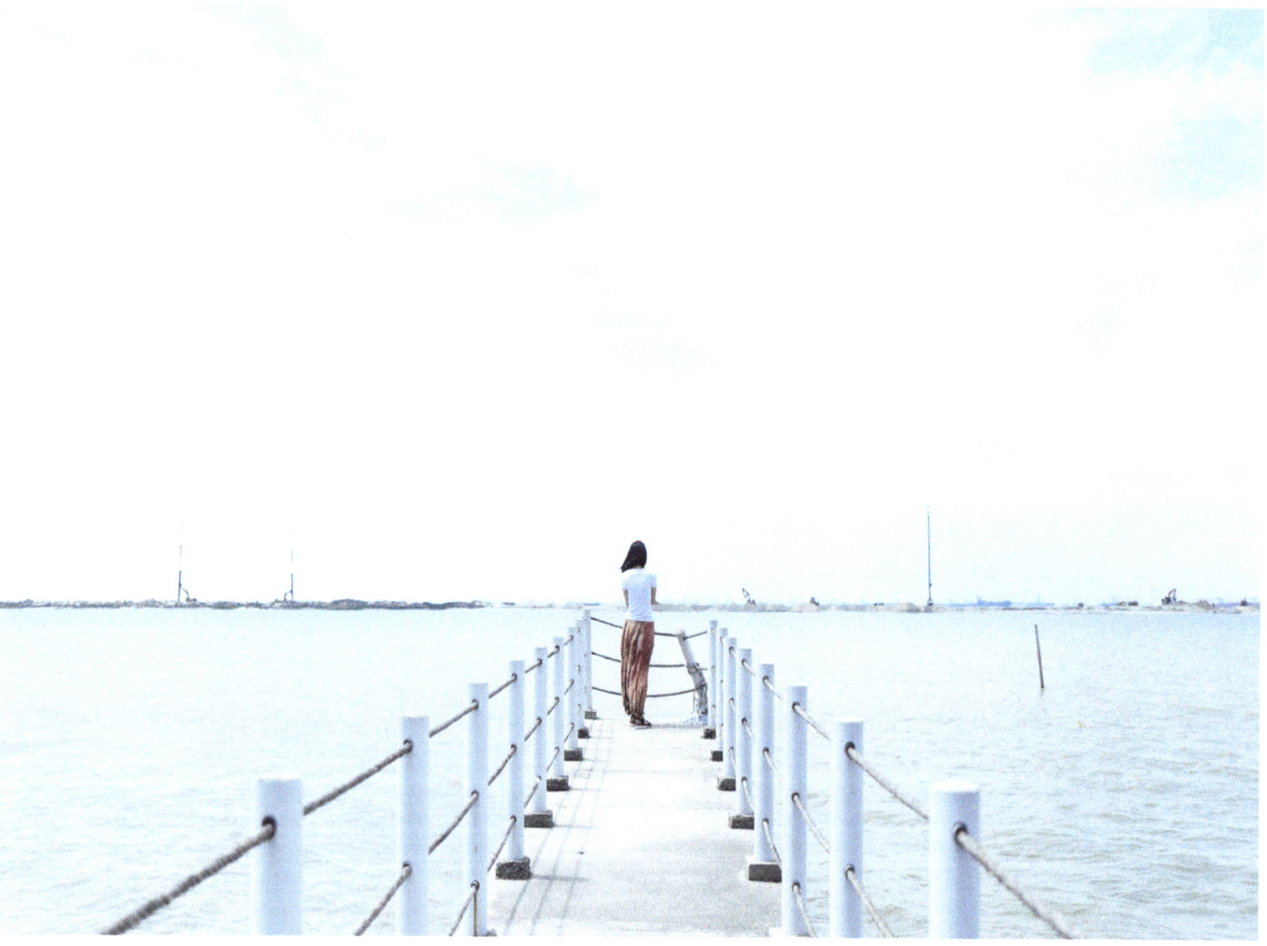

Peace and Harmony within yourself and with the ones that surround you.

Be a Giver instead of a Taker.

Then tomorrow you could be closer to...

Internal peace and being ready to take the journey, in not allowing the bad feelings and hormones to toxify your body and your well-being, and make you gain weight.

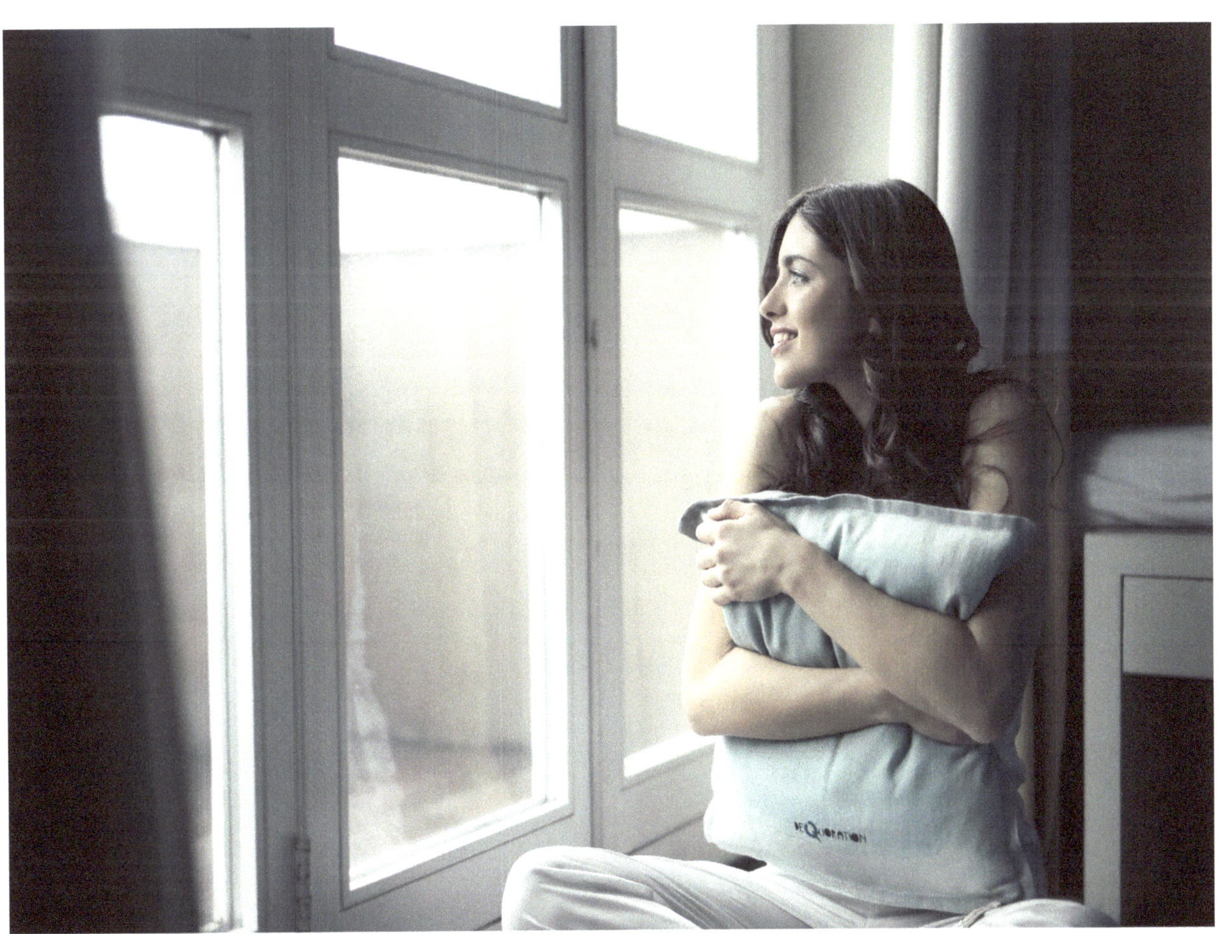

<u>If you are overweight or obese,</u>
<u>*it's not your fault!*</u>

Your DNA played a big role in when and how you became overweight or obese,
Not You!

Your upbringing also played a big part in how you developed your eating's habits,
Not You!

Your level of stress at home and at work also played a big part on how you gained weight,
Not You!

Your emotions and the way you naturally handle life situations, also played a role on how you gained weight,
Not You!

The way your brain controls what you eat and when you eat, plays a daily role on how you gained and keep gaining weight,
Not You!

Health, mental issues, and medications can contribute to your weight gain,
Not You!

Your Brain wants you fat; make no mistake about it!

By now you should have a very good idea, that there are TWO in you: Your SOUL and your BRAIN.

Your BRAIN controls your stomach, and the only way for you to control your stomach, is by you controlling your BRAIN first; there is no other way.

Your Brain wants you to be eating just like the other people that are not losing weight; very logical...

If you lose weight rapidly and your BRAIN finds out; guess what? It wants everything back and more!

The only way to control your BRAIN is to treat it as an adversary that wants to conquer you, the SOUL.

The SOUL is more powerful than the BRAIN when it wants to take over, it can discipline and control the BRAIN, but it's not easy.

THE ONLY PEOPLE THAT ARE SUCESSFUL IN LOSING WEIGHT AND KEEPING IT OFF, ARE THE PEOPLE THAT UNDERSTAND HOW TO CONTROL AND DISCIPLINE THEIR BRAIN.

You must wake up the warrior within you!

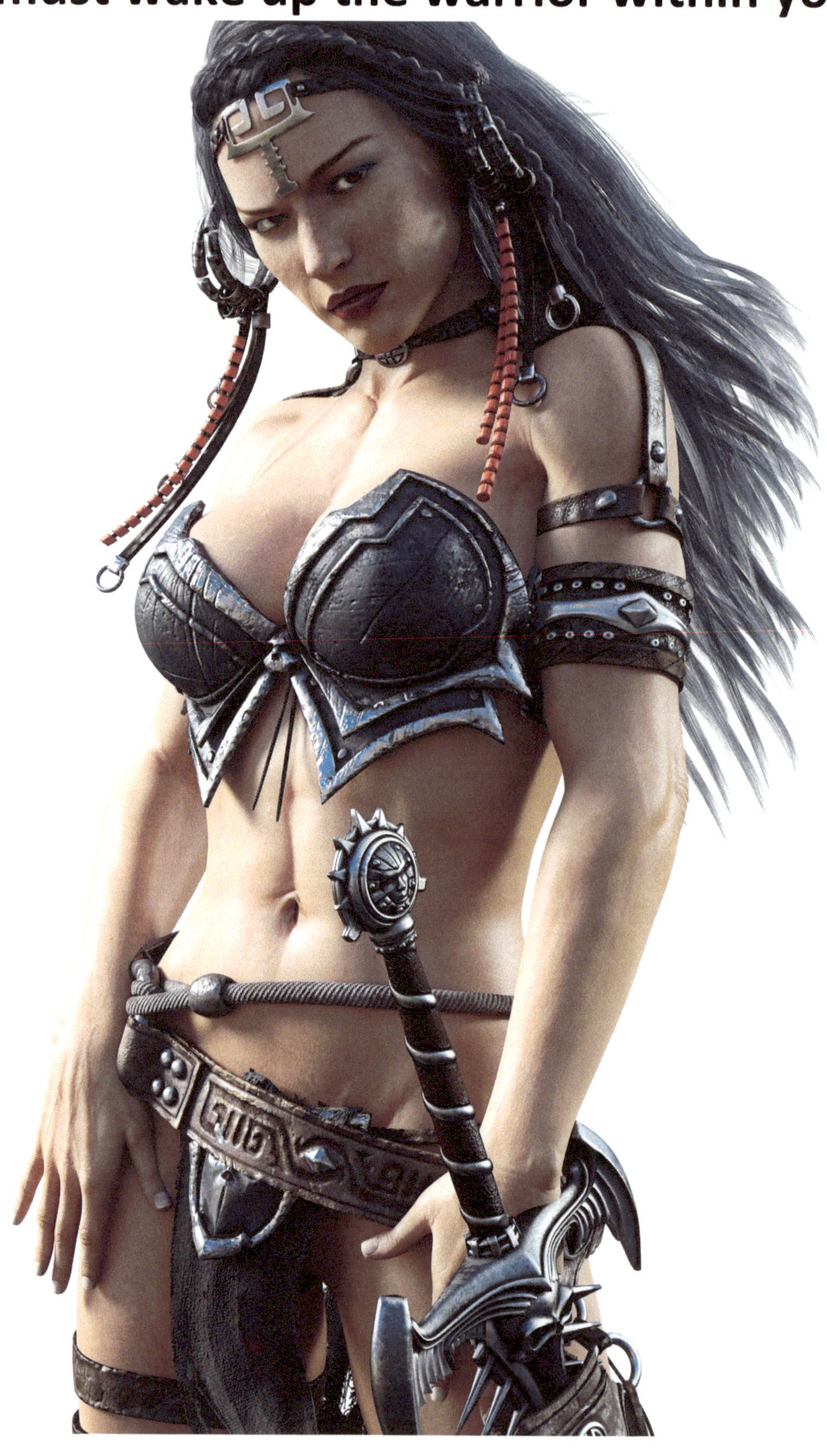

Then, only then, you will be able to control and discipline your own BRAIN!

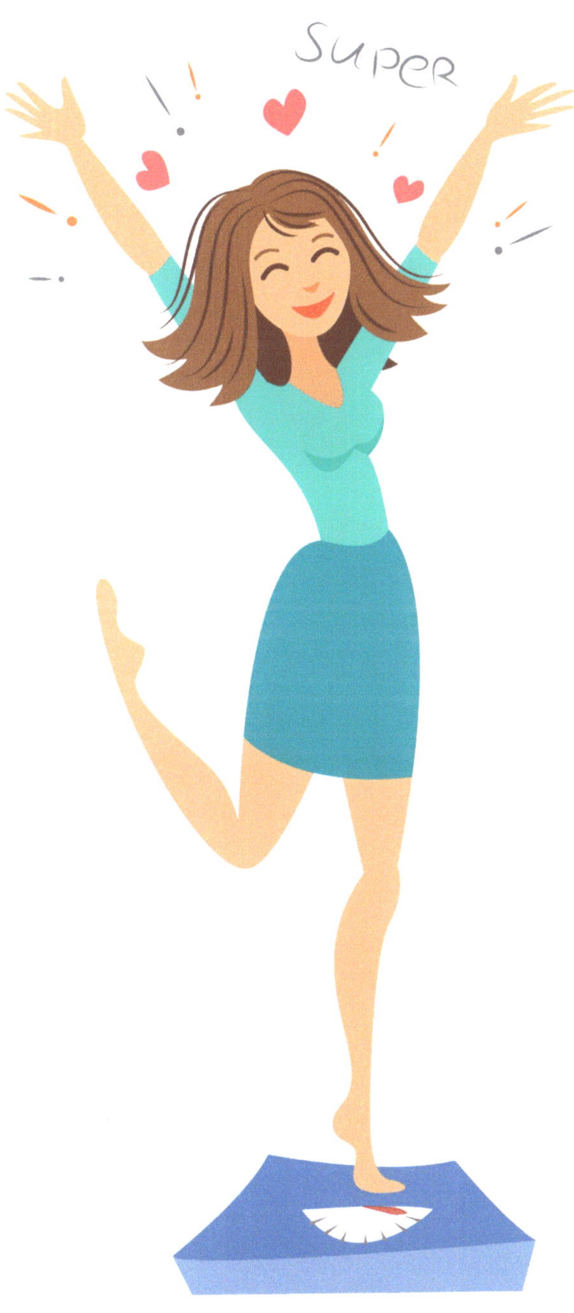

Step on the scale every morning...

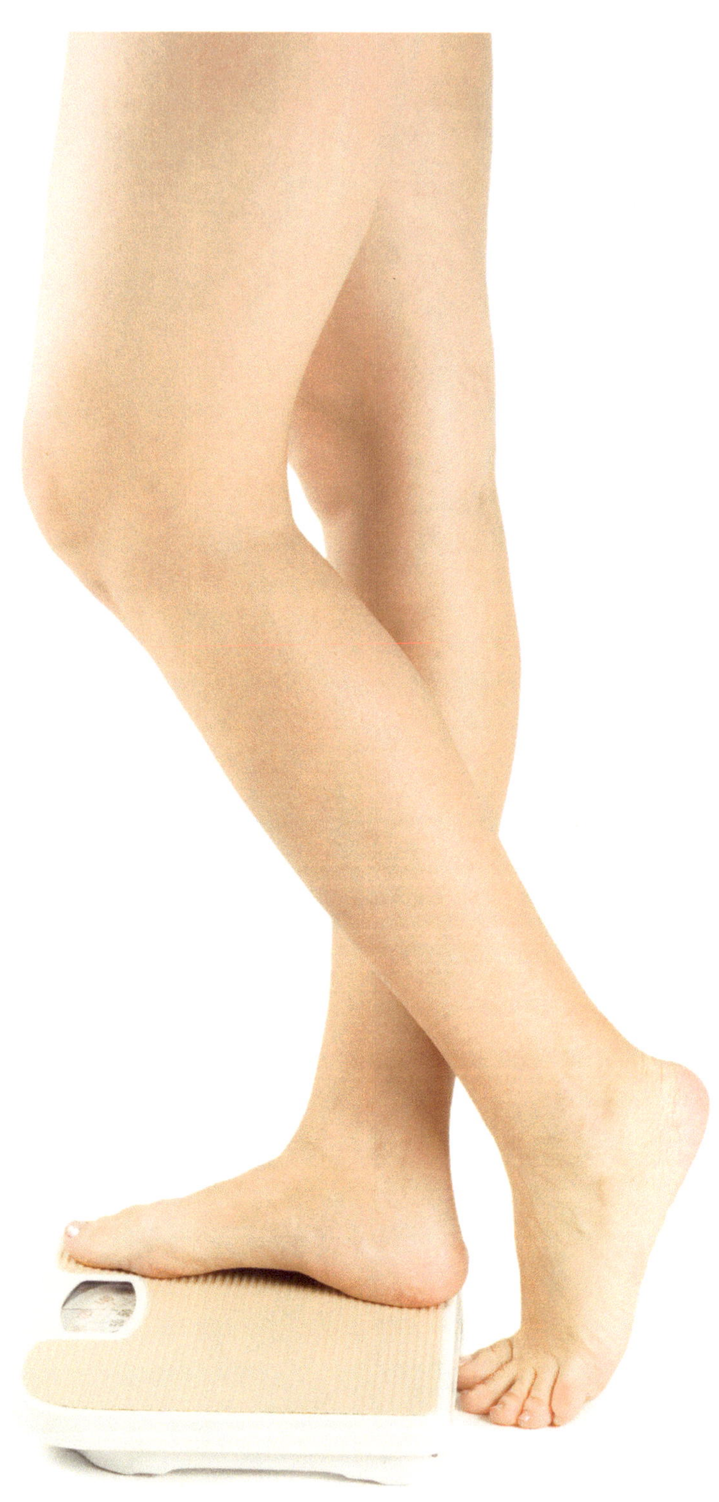

There is no better tool and no better ally than the scale!

It tells you where you were yesterday and where you are today.

It tells you what is working and what is not.

It tells you the truth like no other.

Invest in quality Probiotics and Vitamins

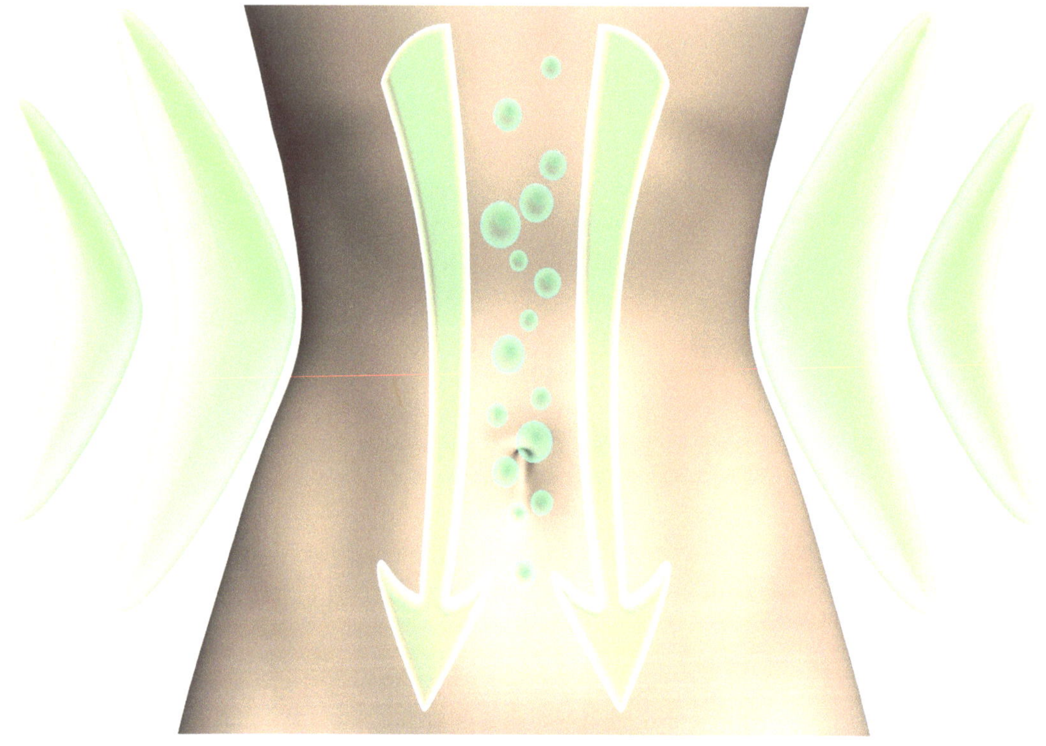

Keep it simple!

Then tomorrow you could be closer...

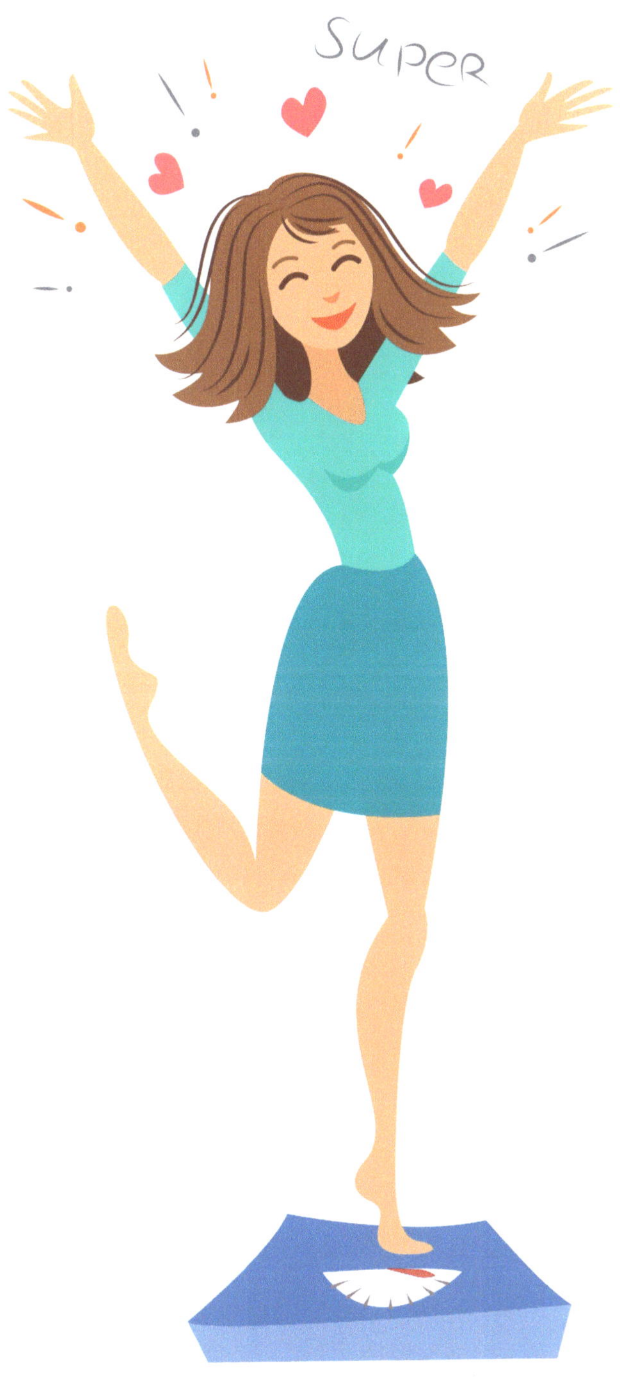

See your health advisor every year!

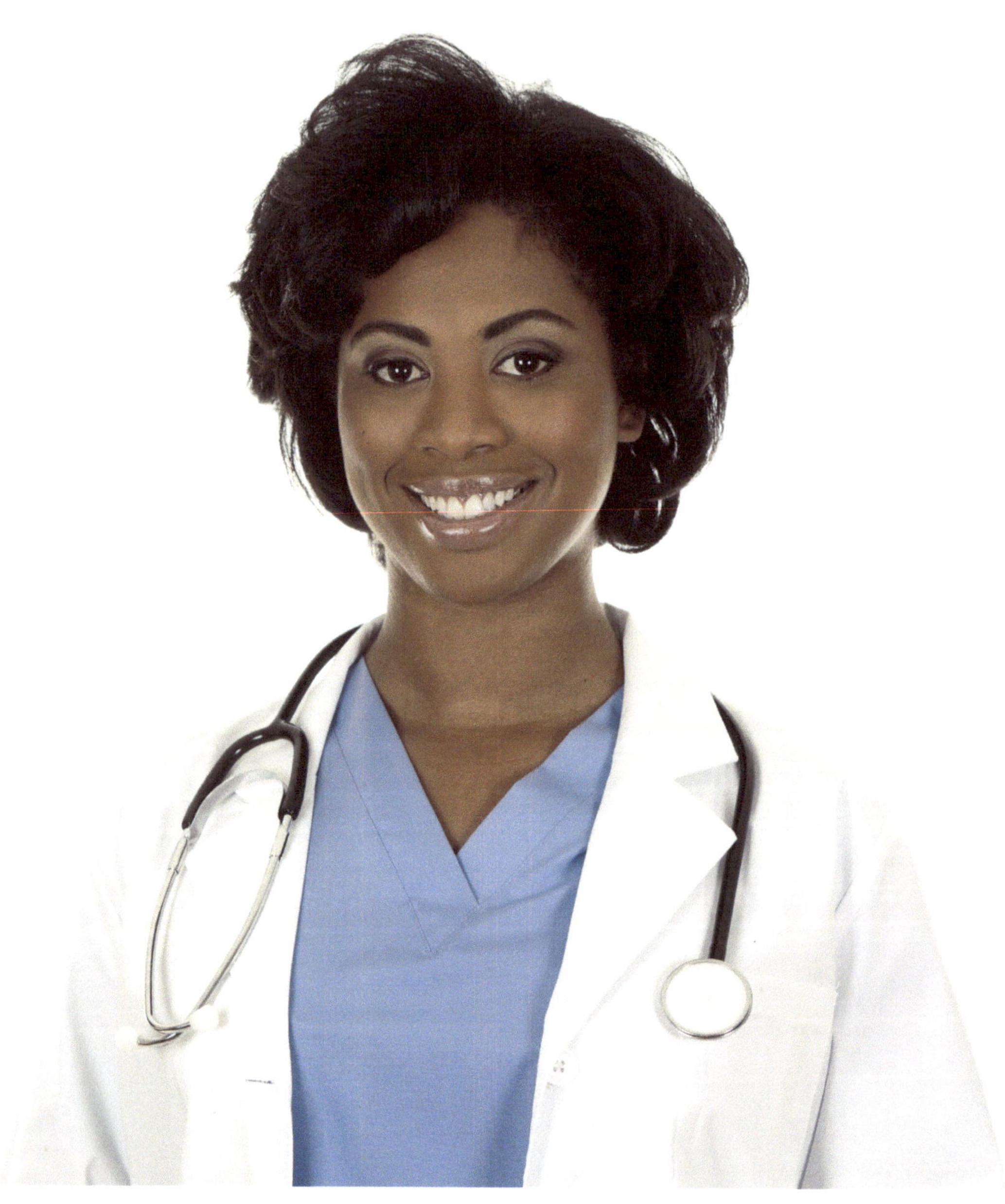

It's your body, the only one you have!

Seeing a doctor at least once a year and before starting any diet is a great move!

Yearly visits can help you manage your health better and can prevent complications in the future.

Go and see someone you feel comfortable with, and that you trust.

Someone that you feel comfortable asking questions, and that is giving you the extra time you need.

If you eat bread and WHEAT products...

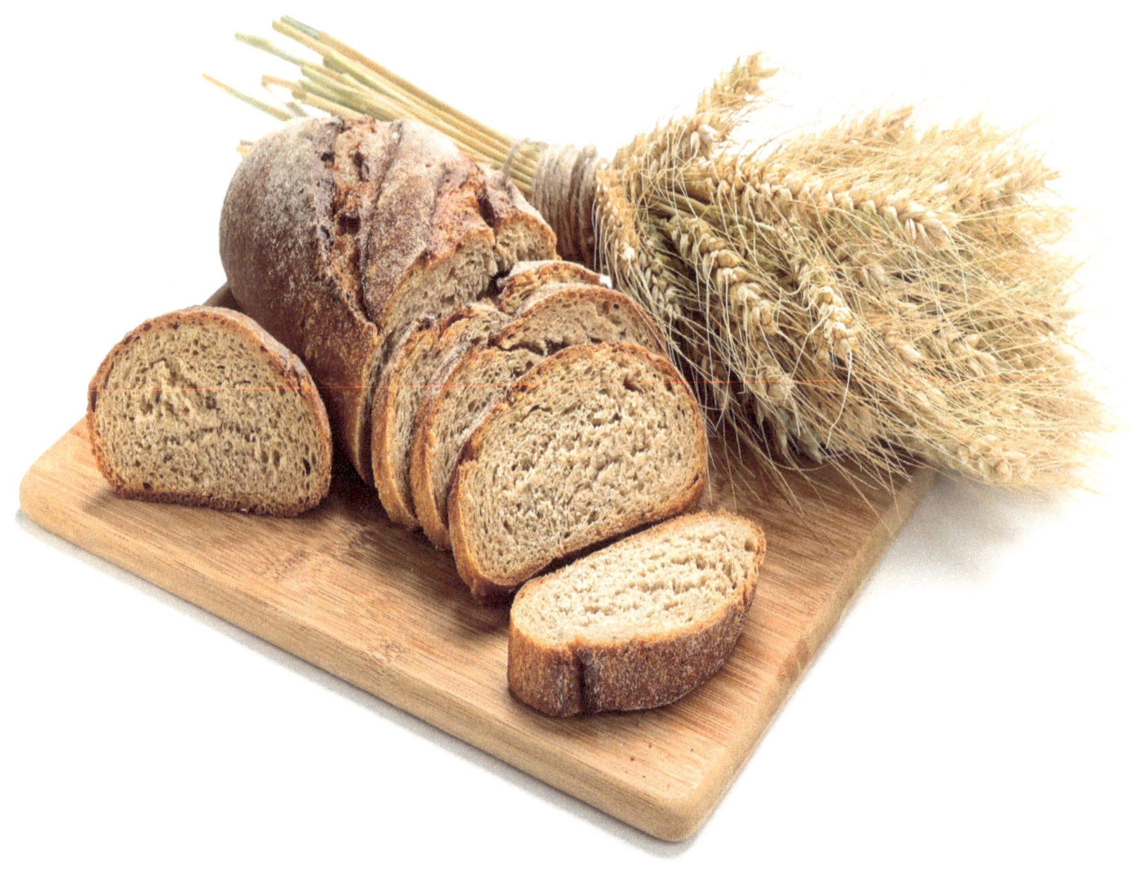

(YOUR #2 ENEMY)

Then tomorrow you could be closer to...

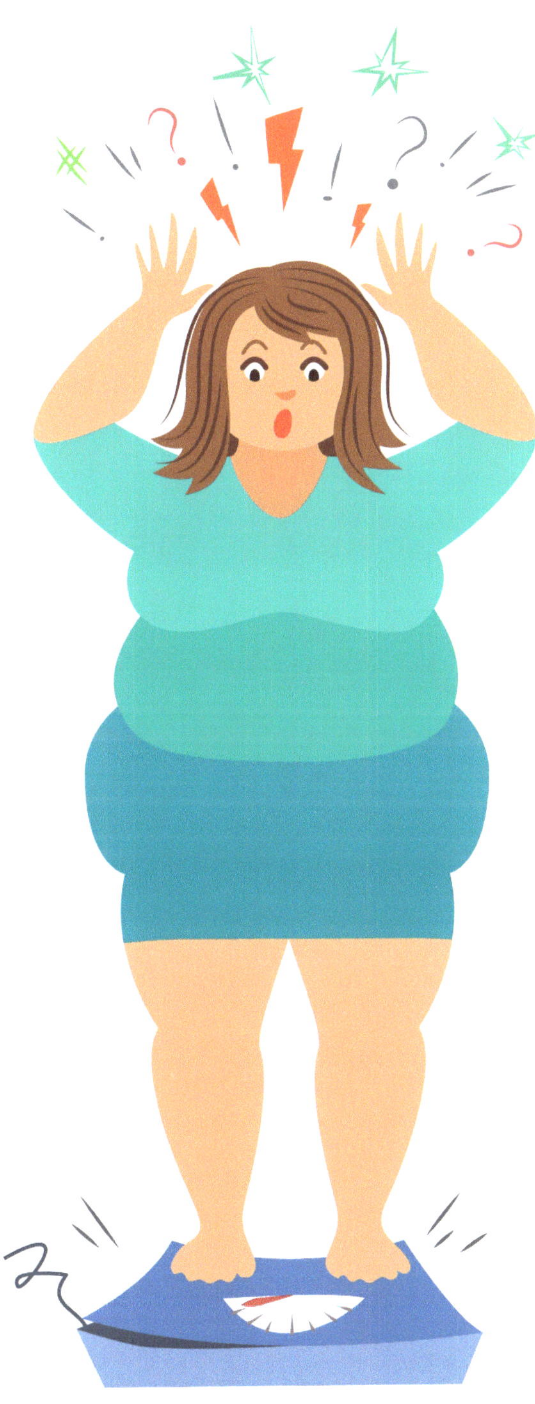

<u>Most effective way to reduce Belly Fat!</u>

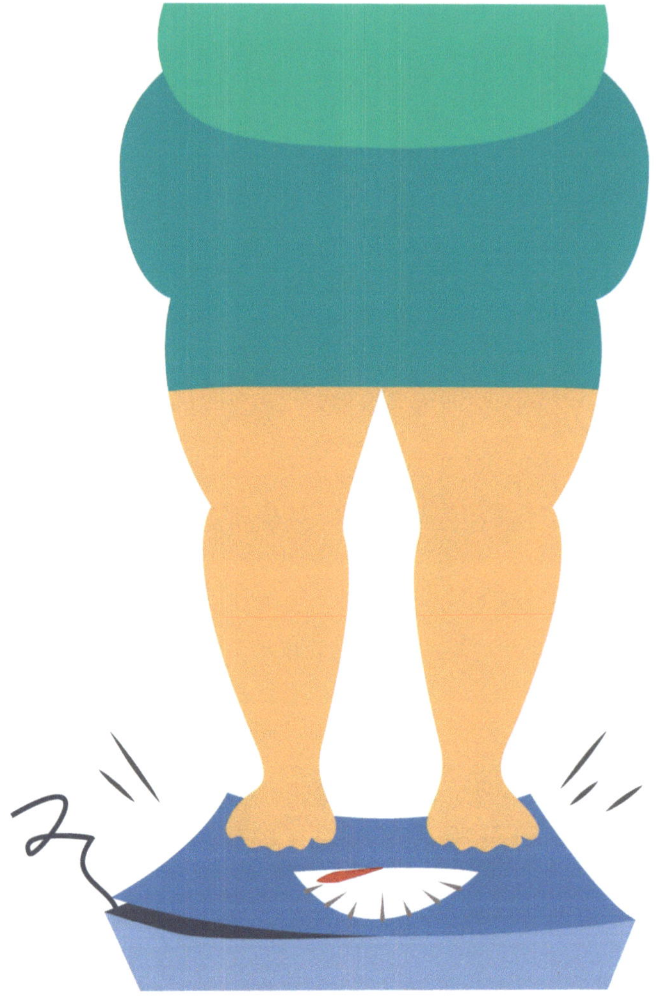

Eat no more than 30g of Carbohydrate for 10 or more consecutives days.

The more days you eat less than 30g of carbohydrates the more belly fat you will lose.

Drink plenty of water!

You govern yourself; nobody else!

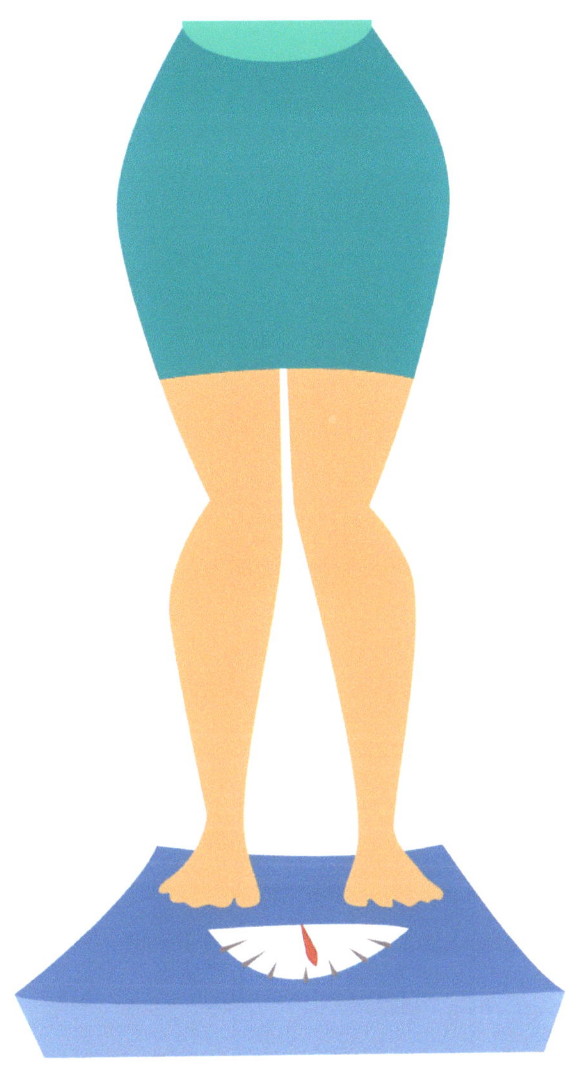

If you eat meat today...

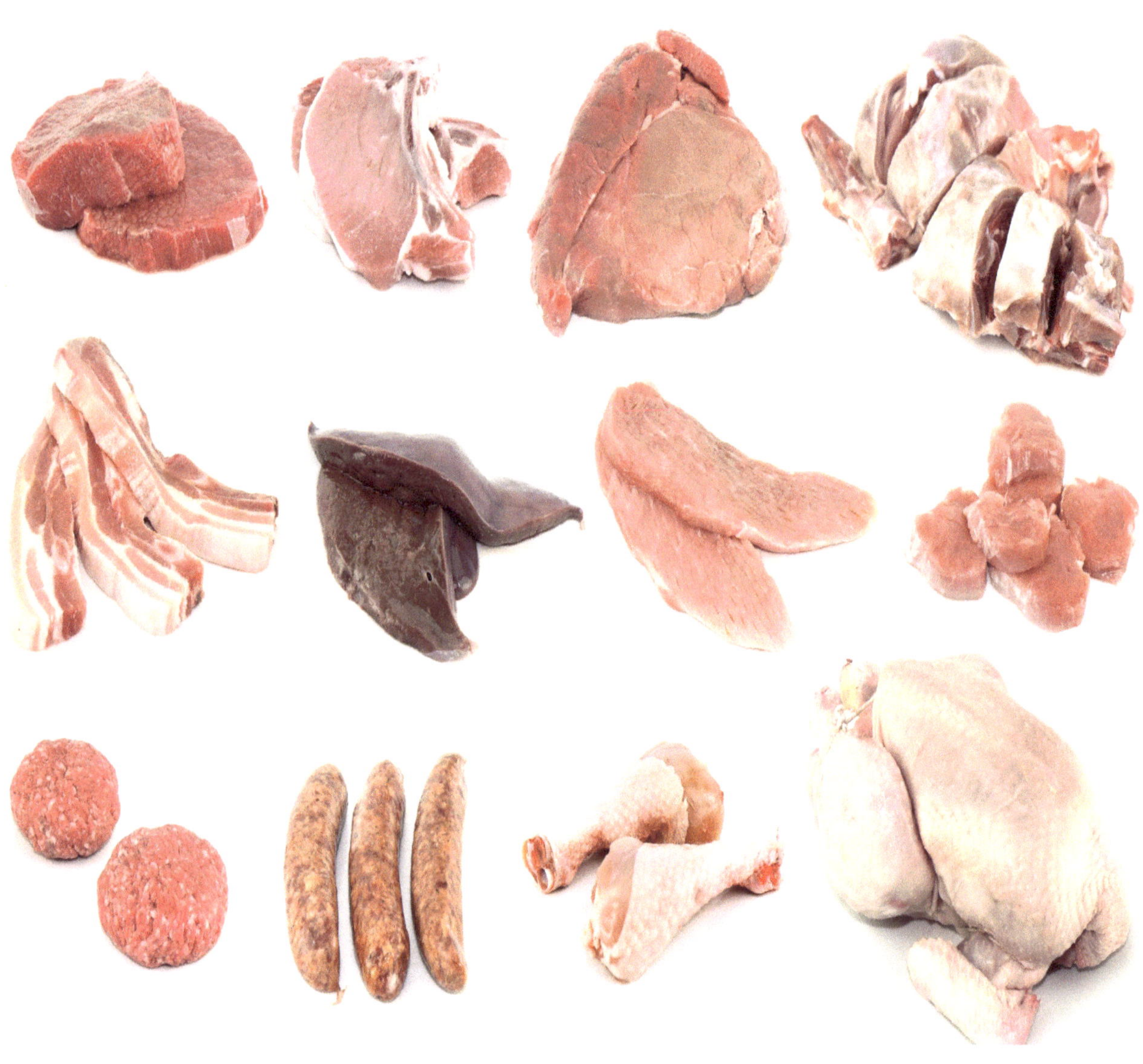

Then tomorrow you could be closer to

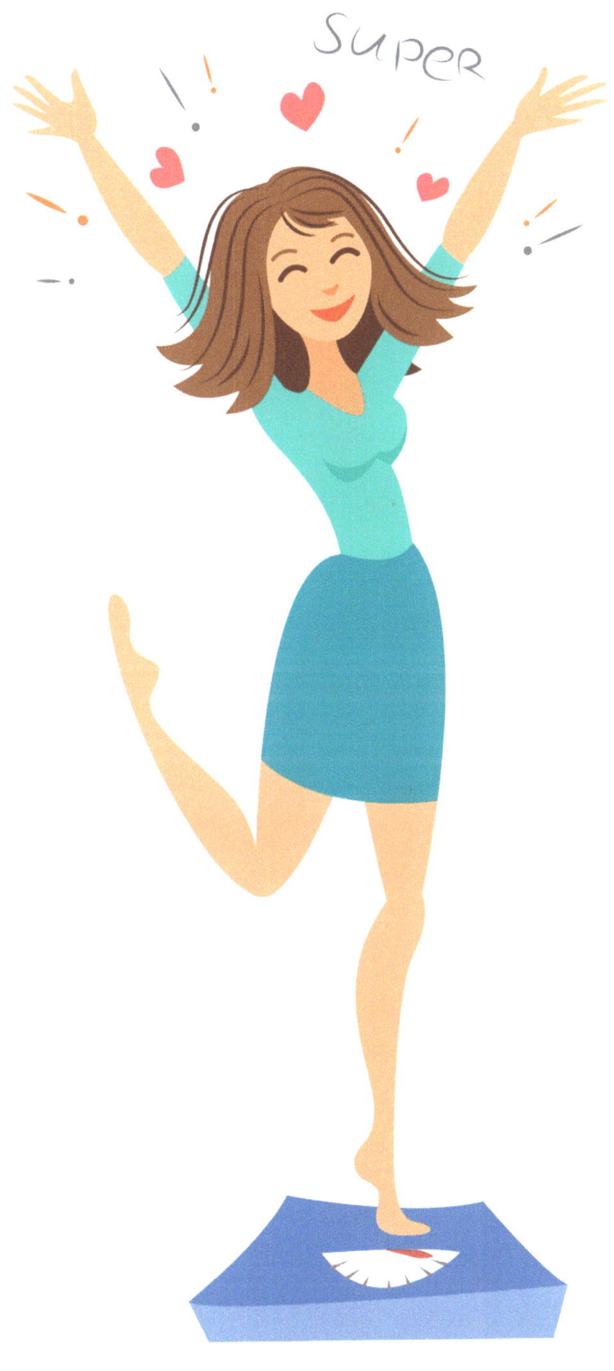

If you eat pasta today...

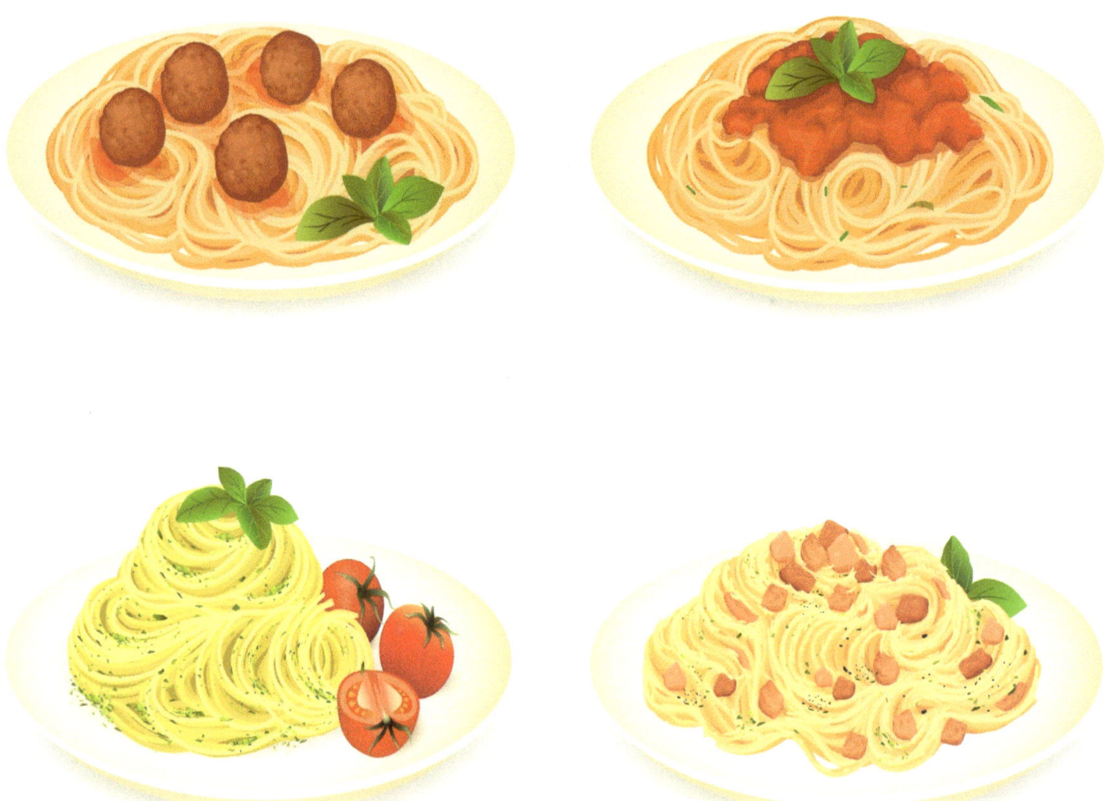

Then tomorrow you could be closer to…

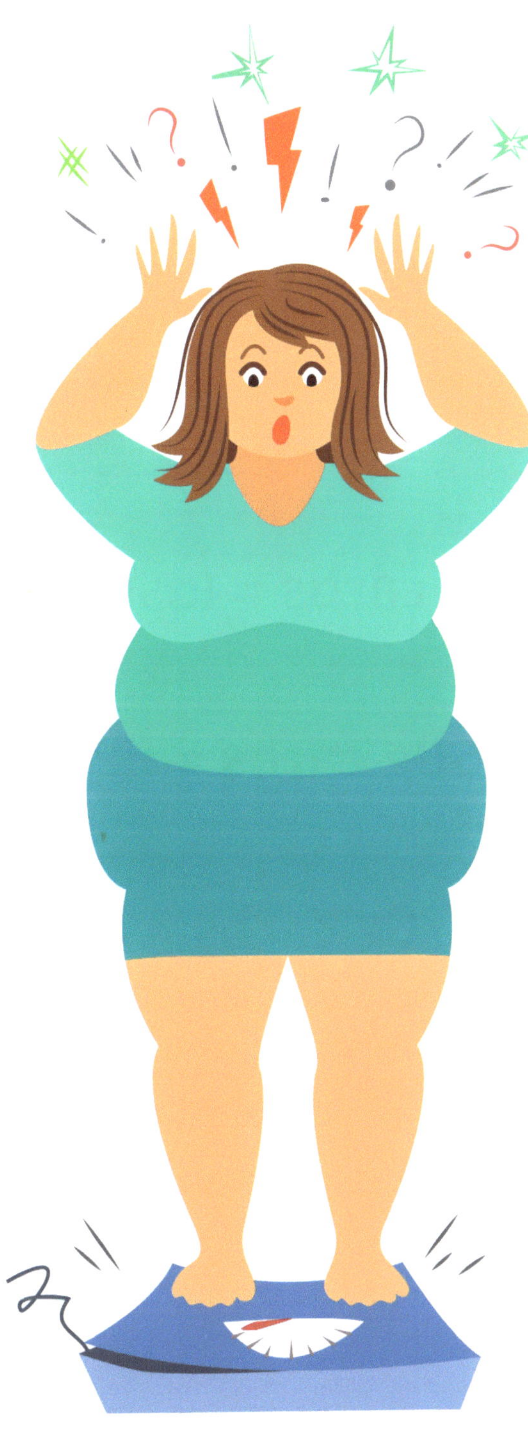

My little simple table that works!

If your intake for many CONSECUTIVES days of carbohydrates are:

Less than 30g carbs = losing lots of weight

Between 30-50g carbs = losing little weight

Between 50-70g carbs = losing no weight

Over 70g carbs = gaining proportional to the intake of carbs.

YOUR DAILY choice!

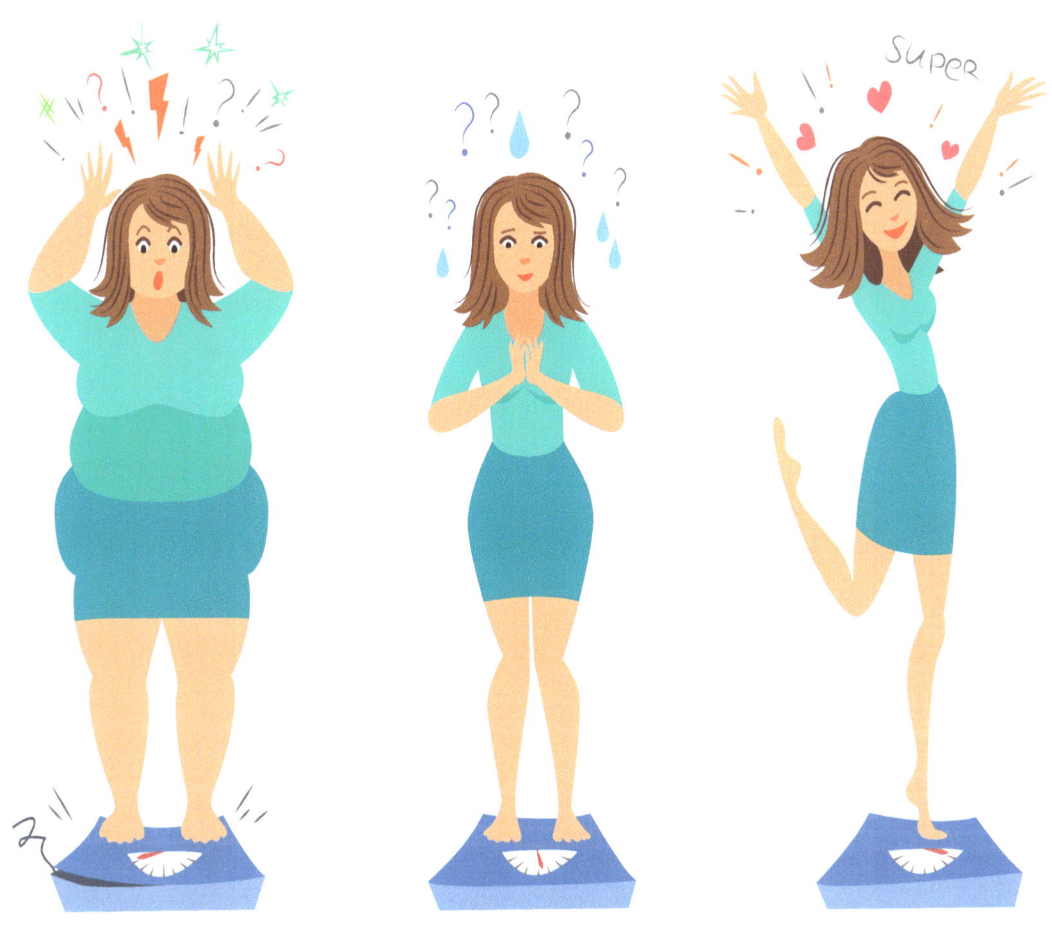

IT'S YOUR BODY!

If you eat vegetables today...

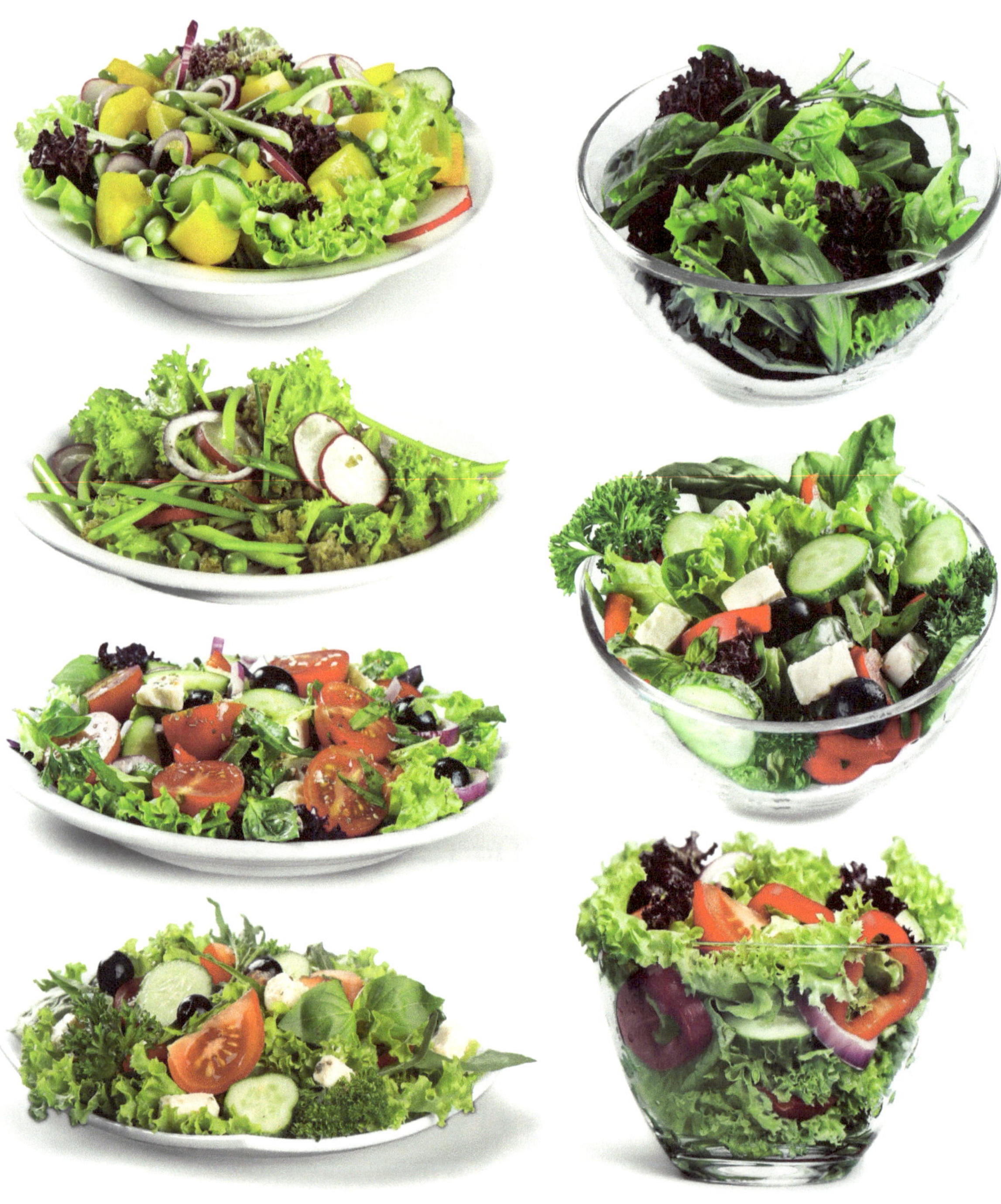

Then tomorrow you could be closer to...

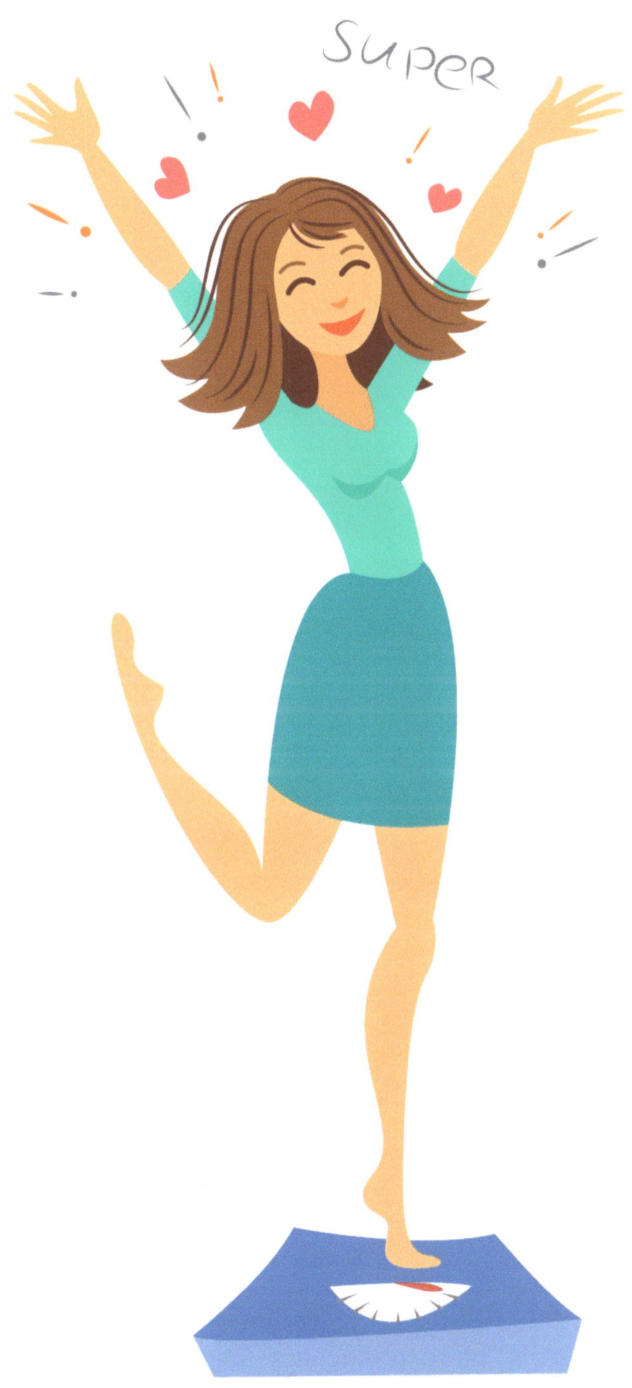

If you eat sweets today...

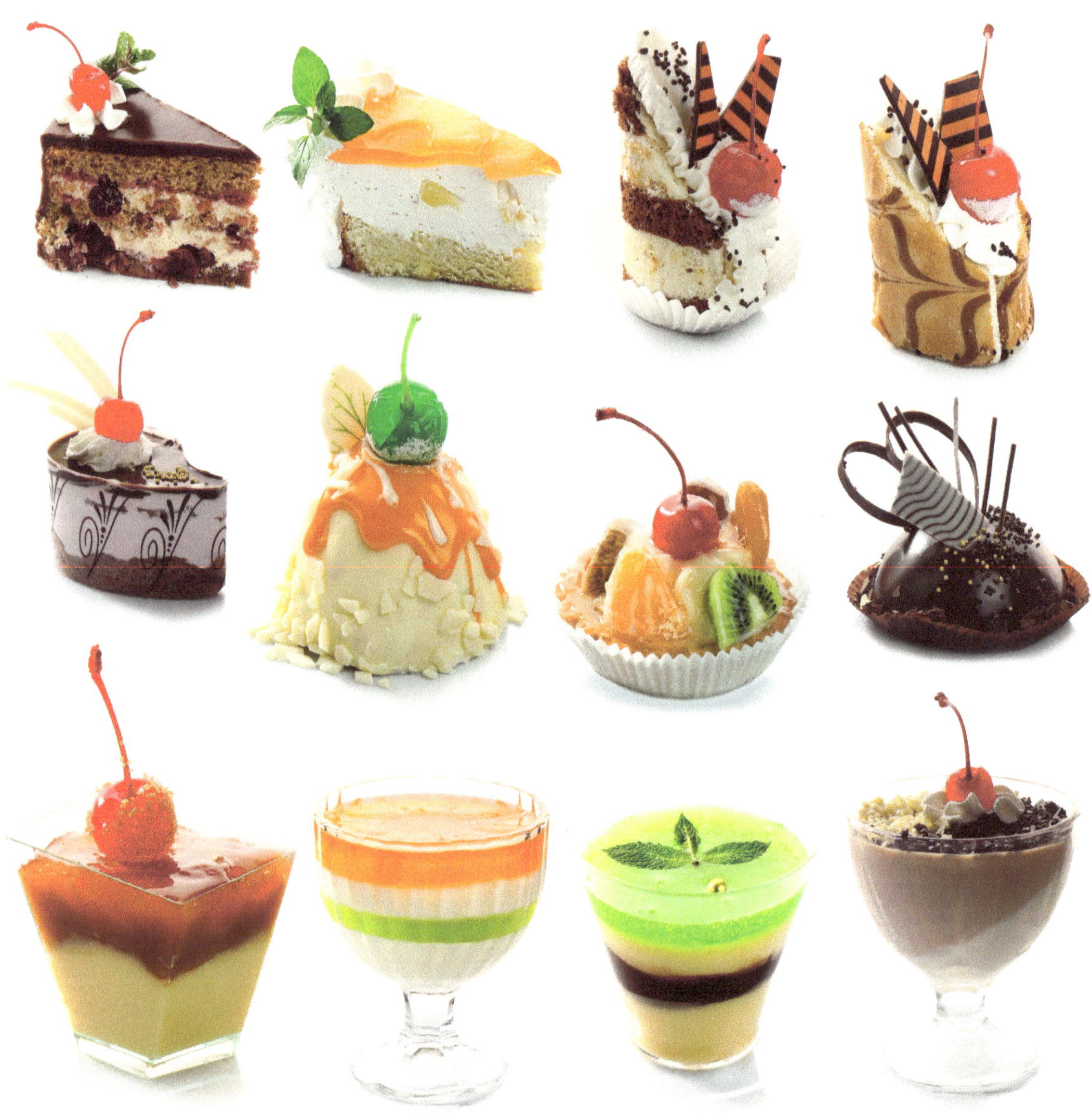

(YOUR #1 ENEMY)

Then tomorrow you could be closer to...

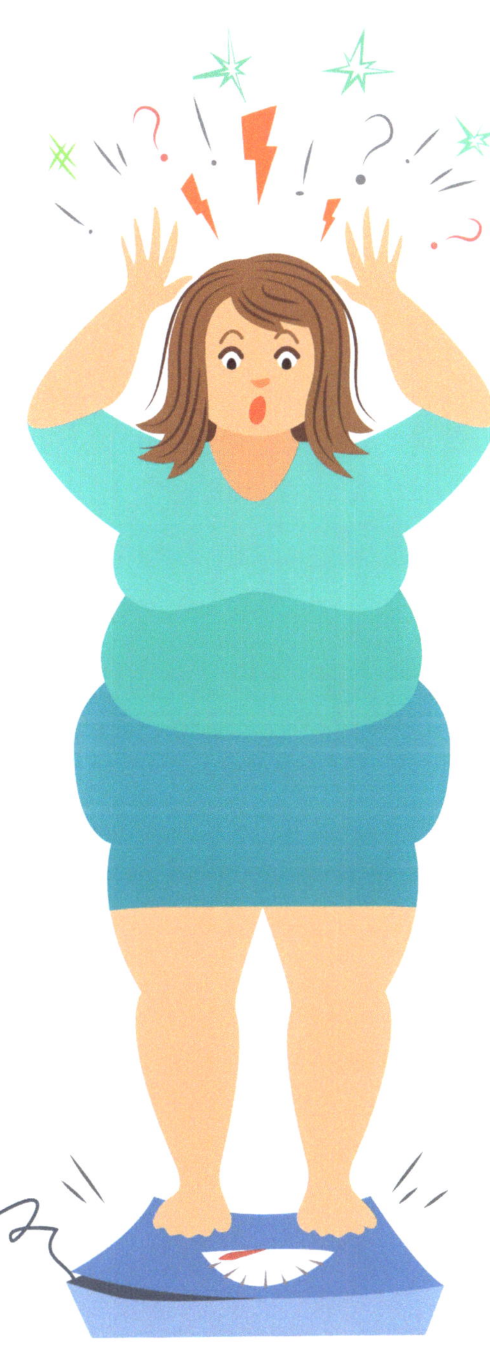

If you exercise today...

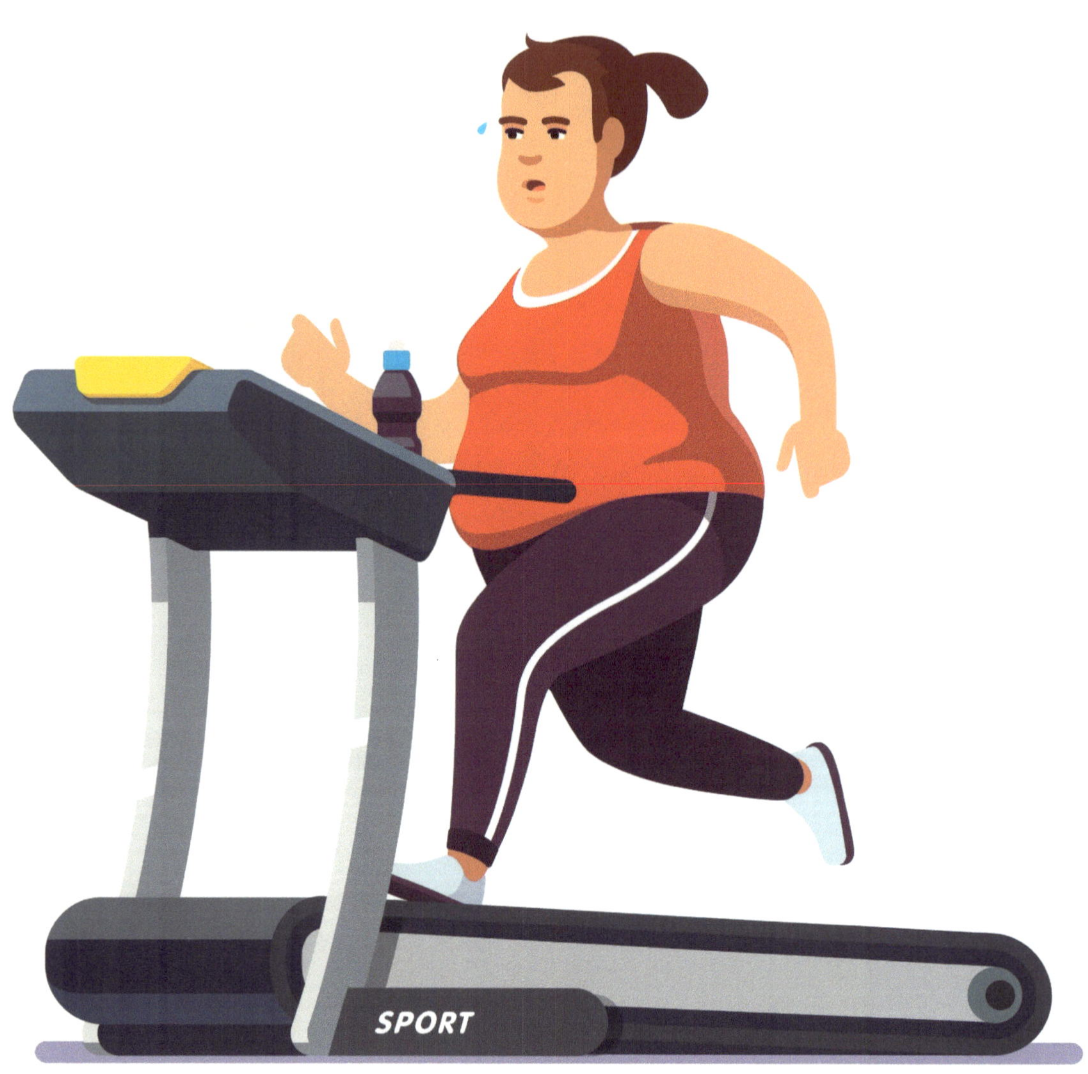

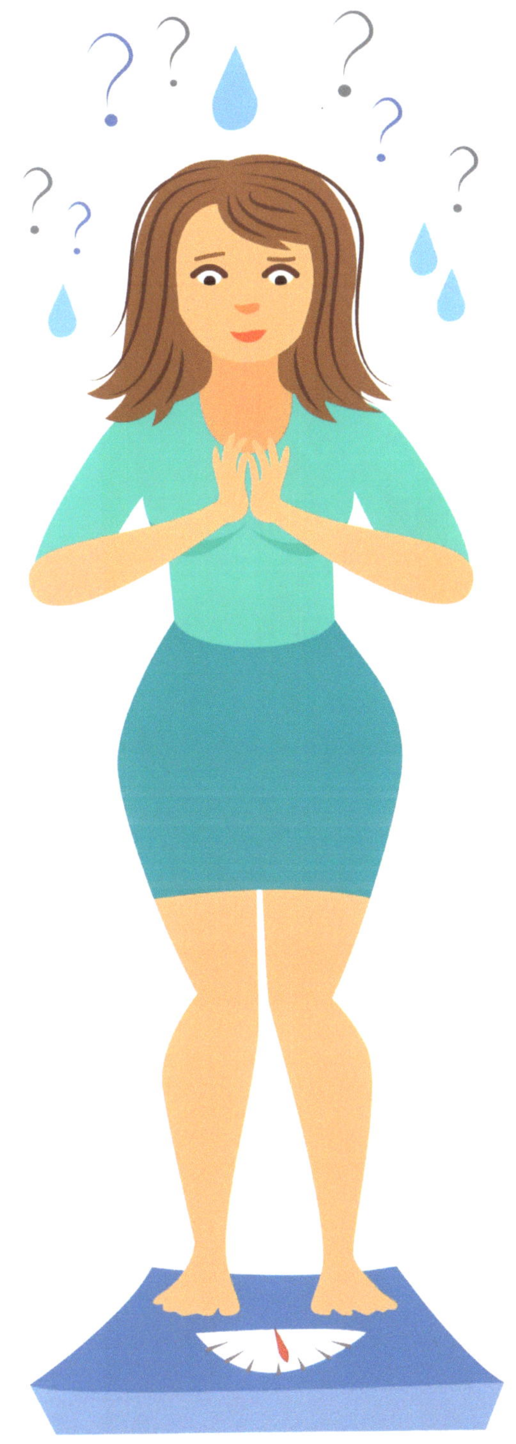

Exercise doesn't really help as much as we think when it comes to losing weight.

A lot of it
has to do with
eating the
right food to help
you lose
the extra weight.

Exercise can make you hungry and you could end up eating more.

Move and walk naturally as much as you desire.

If you eat fish today...

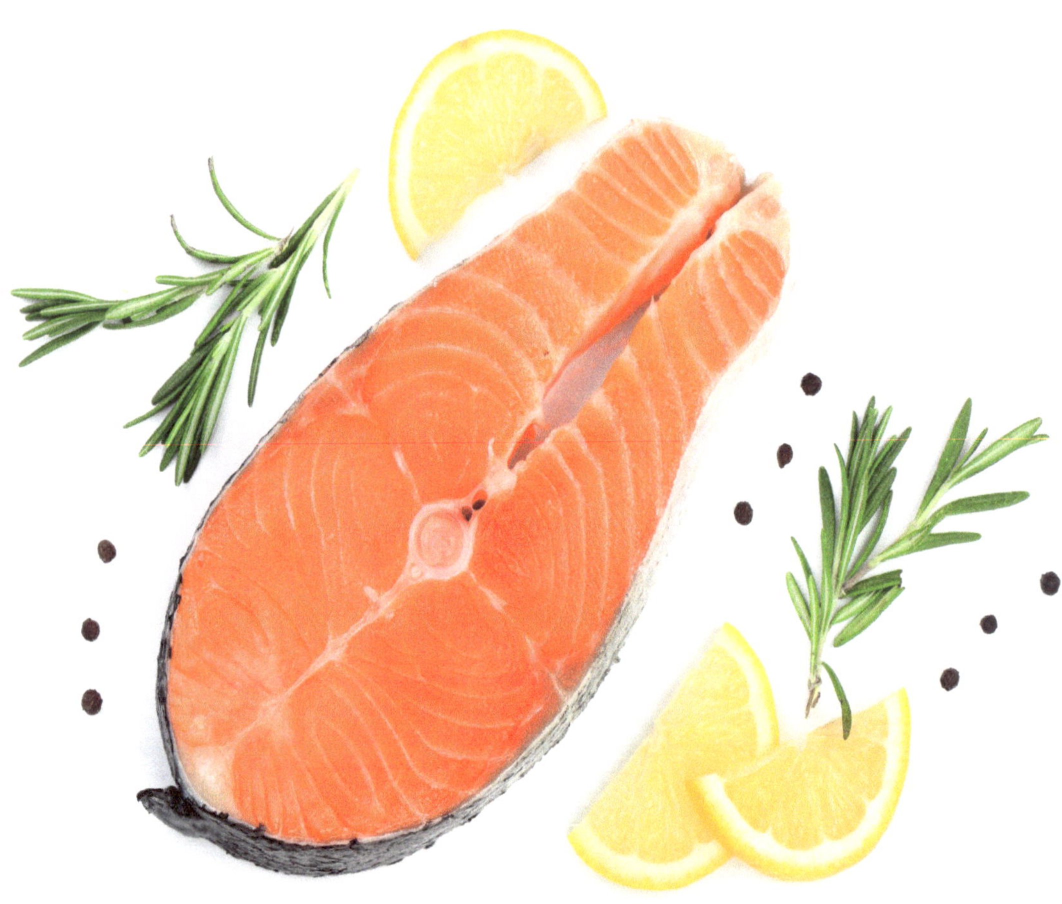

Then tomorrow you could be closer to...

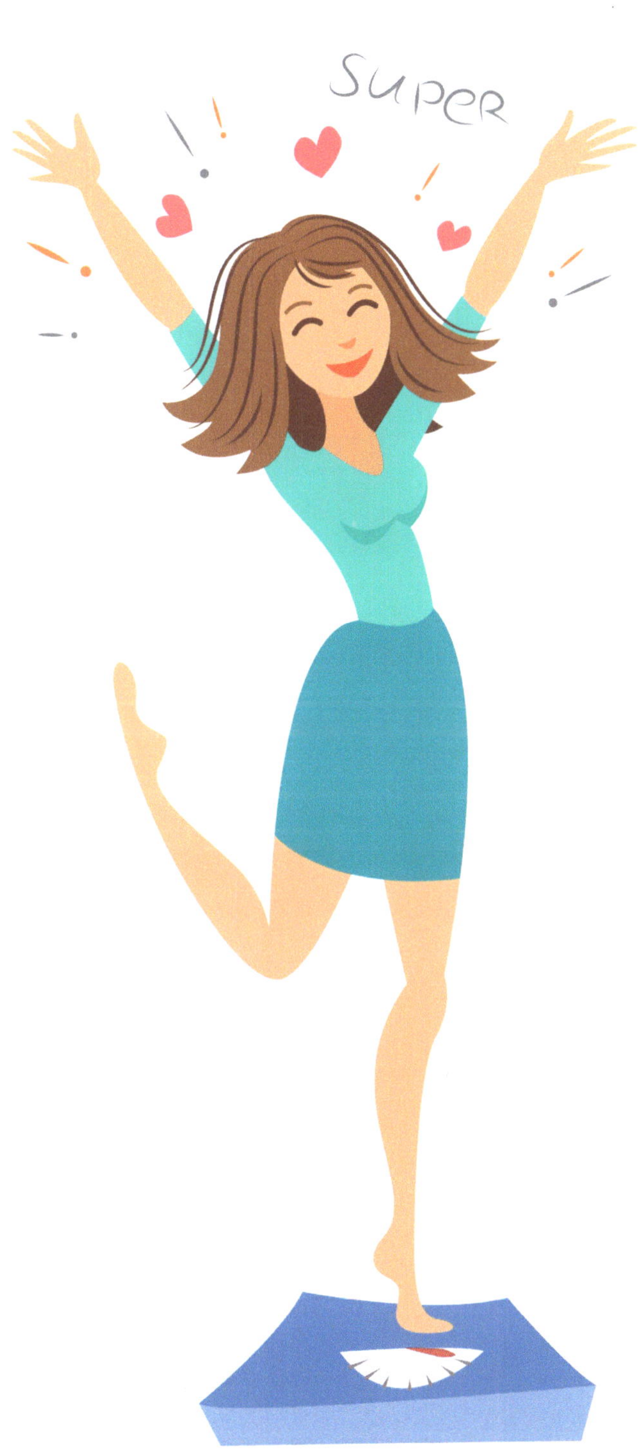

<u>Cheat once in while!</u>

Yes. Replace a meal with one, even two cups of ice cream, or a slice, or maybe two slices of pizza, or anything you want.

Why not?

The key is to do it very sporadically. And once you do it, go back on track and don't cheat for a few days.

And when you get into the cycle of cheating/"failure" for more than 2 days, keep weighing yourself. That weight gain will give you the motive to go back to eating right to lose more weight.

My "failures" of gaining back the weight while going off track, gave me the motivation to go back on my diet with a vengeance and lose more weight.

By cheating once in a while, you are creating a WIN-WIN situation with your brain. Especially in the first weeks, if you don't let your brain WIN a few times, your BRAIN will get very upset at you, and will punish you by making you eat more than what you were eating before, and all the weight you have lost, will come back.

Do not attach time frame to a weight loss plan; let it just happen!

Do not set unrealistic goals; let it just happen!

<u>Time to Change the Rules!</u>

Who said that we need to eat three meals a day?

Experiment with skipping breakfast, just coffee with milk, or tea a few times in the morning, drink plenty of water, then start your first meal at 10:30 or 11:00am, eat your second meal at 3 or 4pm, and finish off with a light snack around 7pm.

Experiment with you controlling your own brain, and you, yes you, can tell your brain to direct your stomach to wait a little longer to eat, just like our ancestors, they needed to go and hunt for a few hours and then prepare the meals when they got back. By the time the whole tribe was ready to eat, it was night time; they ate mostly meat and berries.

And they ate one meal, yes, one meal a day!

There were no means to store food, everything was basically eaten in one sitting a day! But we want to do three sittings a day to eat, and sometimes four or more!

Who said that we need to eat on a big full plate?

Get a medium or small plate and learn how to eat half of what you are currently eating. How are you expecting to lose weight if you keep eating the same portions and number of meals as you always have? It does not make sense.

Review and Change what is not working for you.

If you eat too many of these fruits today...

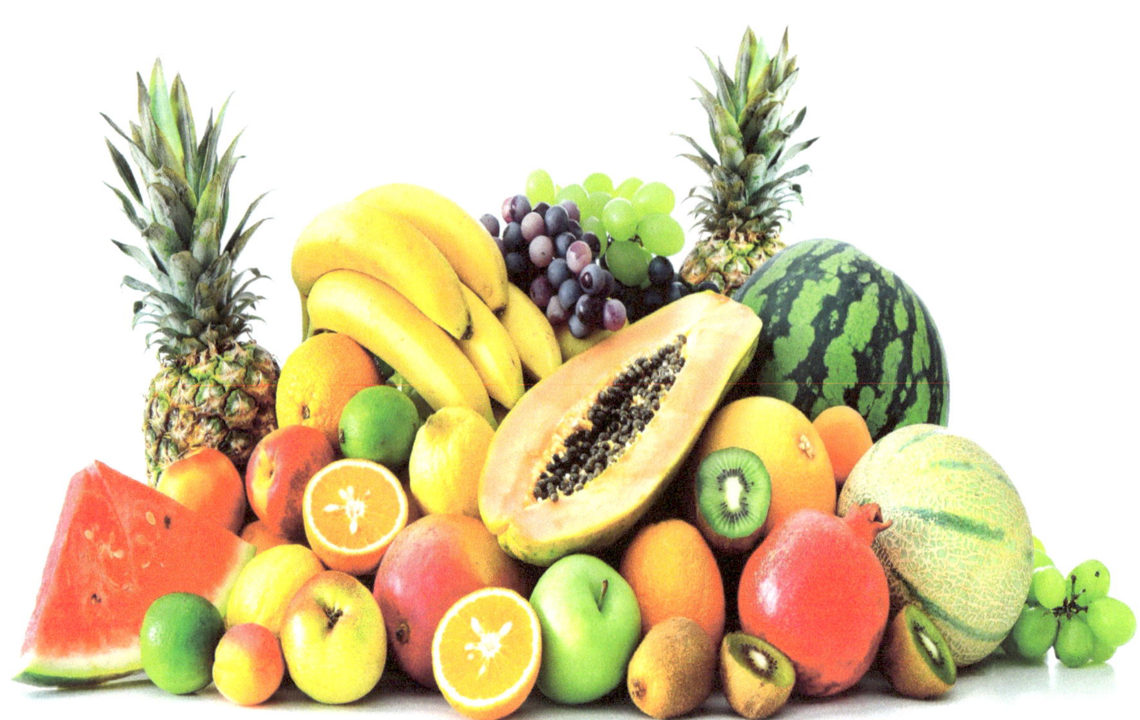

Then tomorrow you could be closer to...

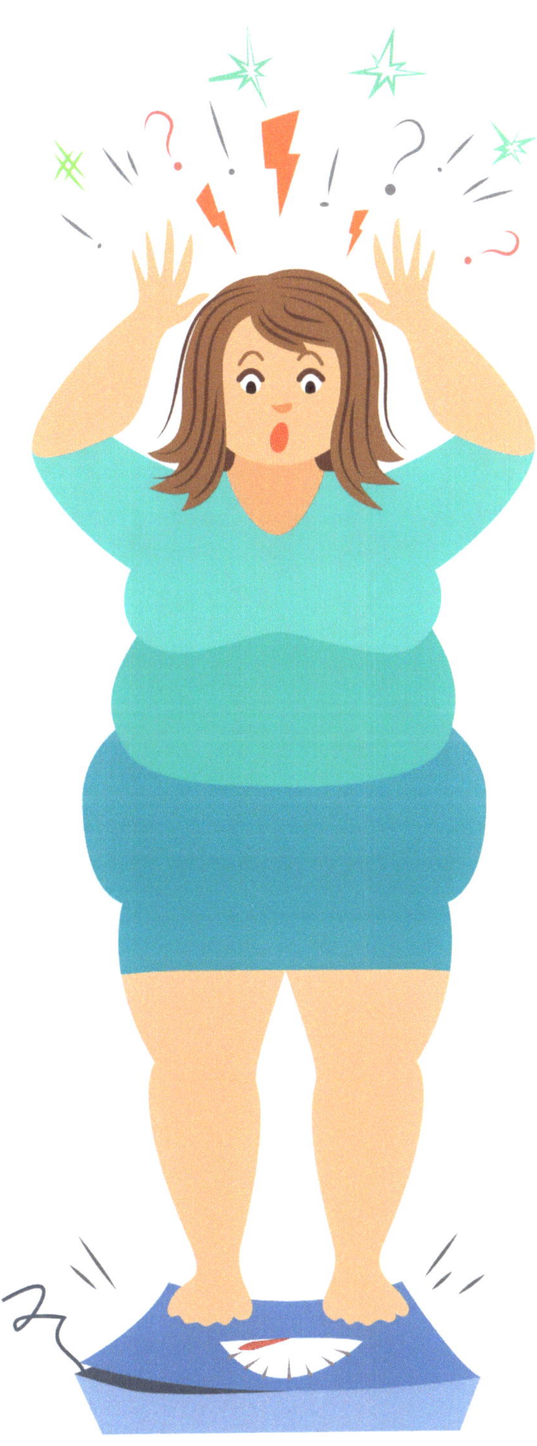

If you eat some berries today...

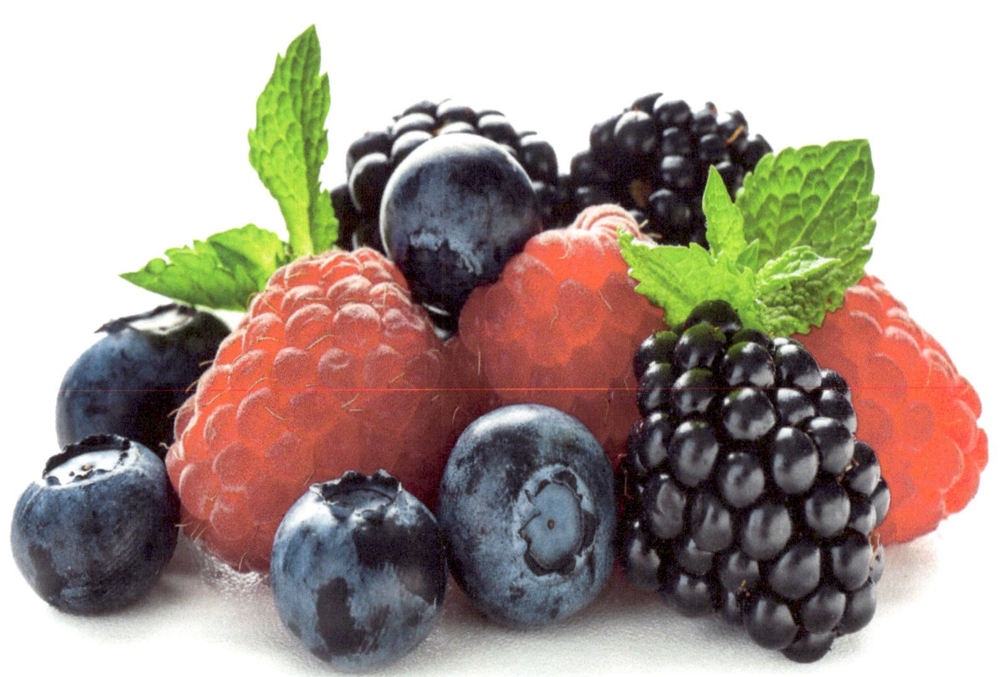

Then tomorrow you could be closer to...

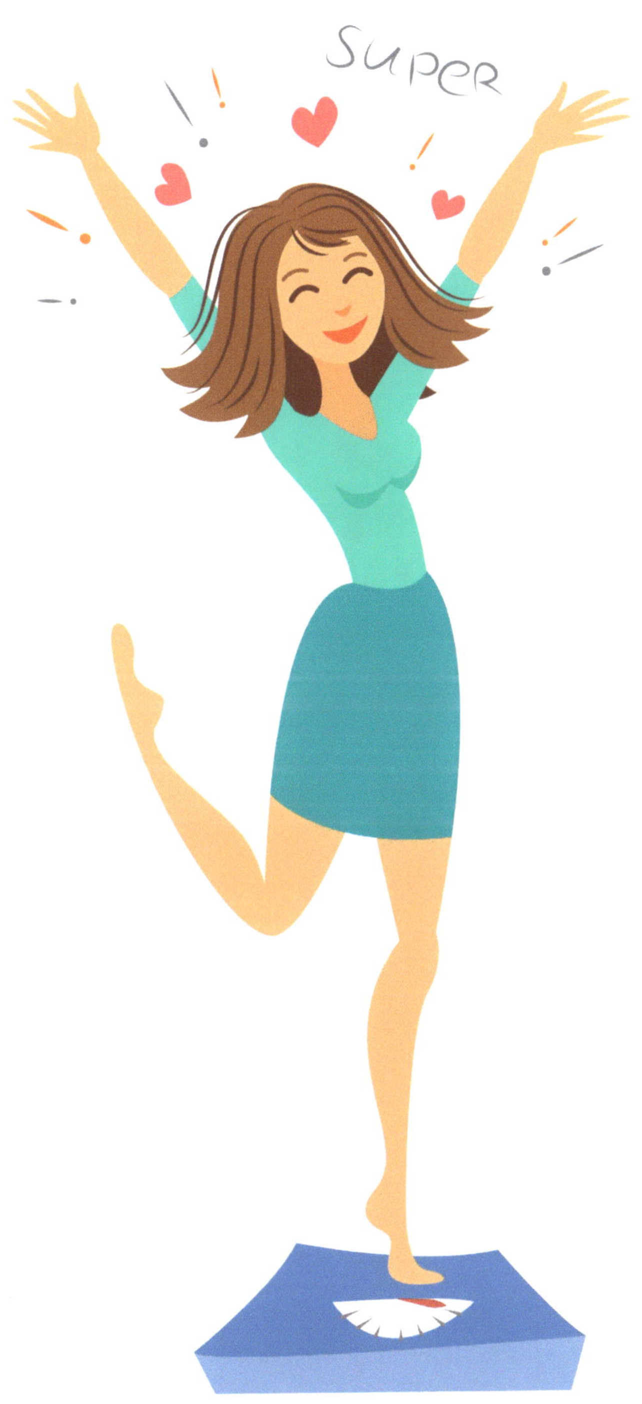

If you drink alcohol today...

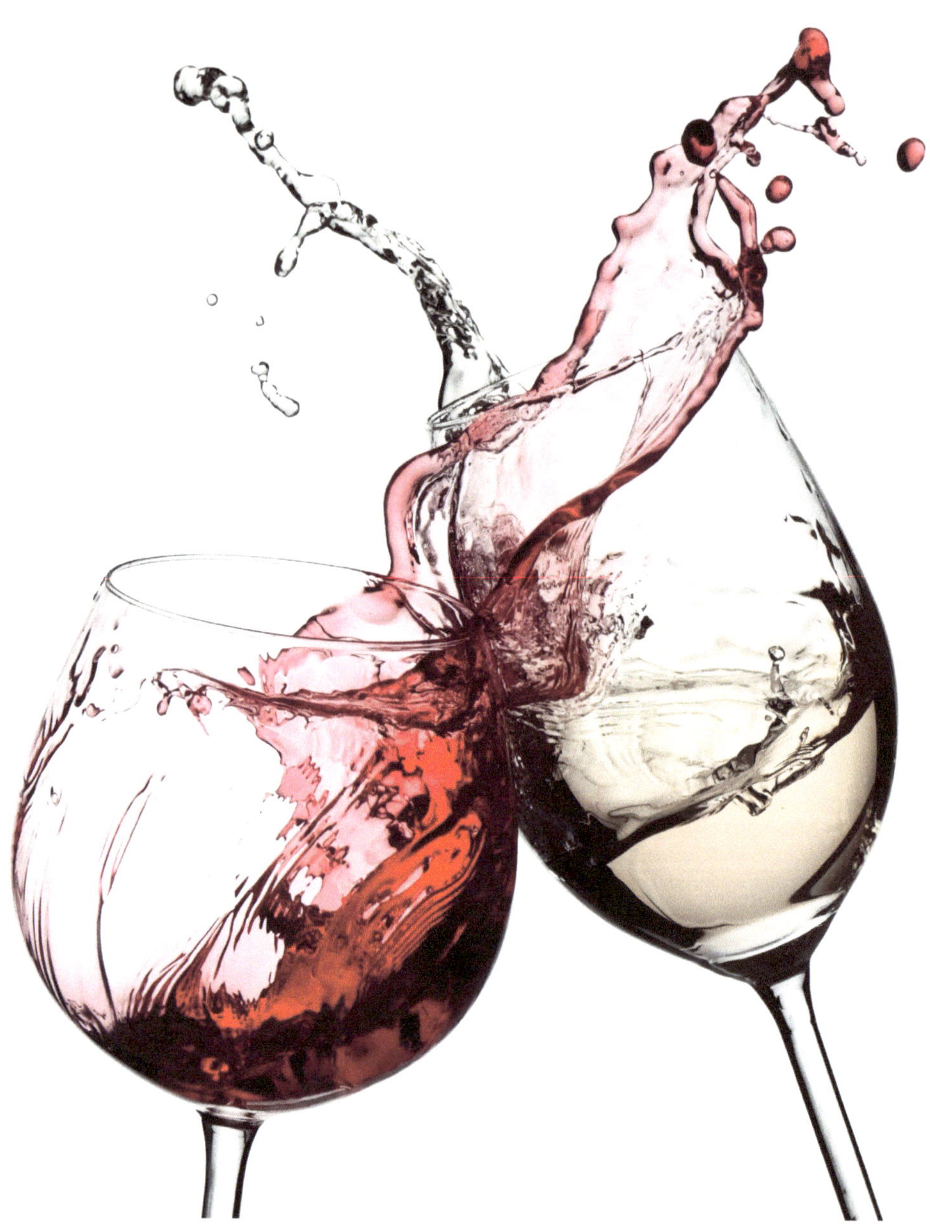

Then tomorrow you could be closer to...

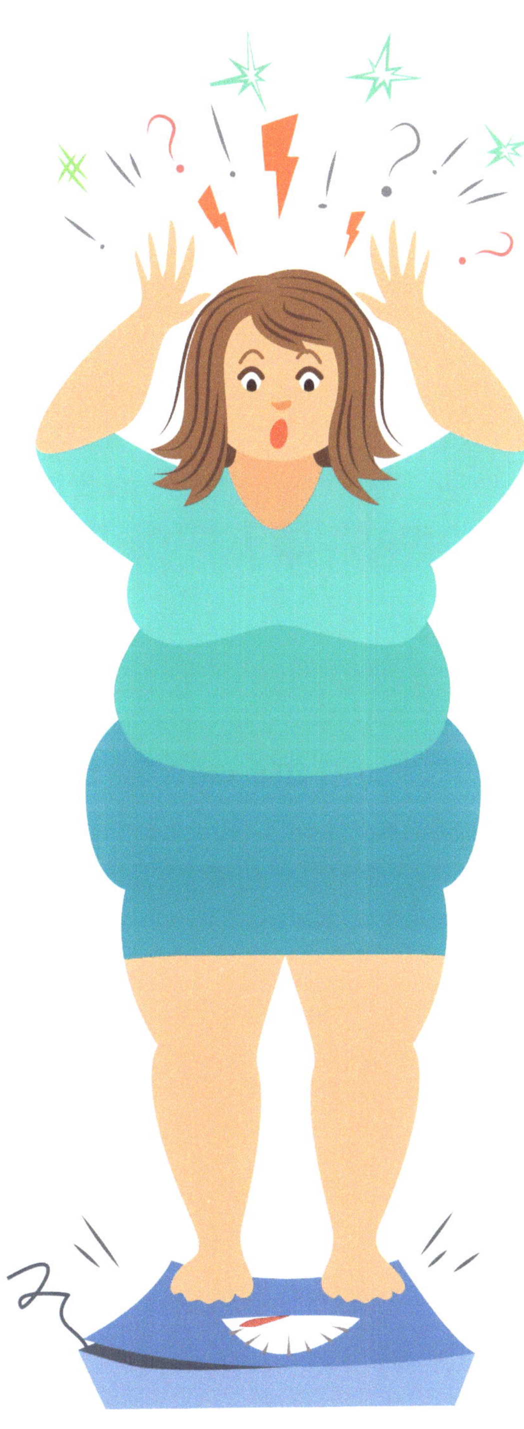

Weight loss is one of the most difficult endeavors that you will undertake in your life.

It is difficult because:

1. You are going against your DNA, or nature, some people would say that it's almost impossible. Nature will always try to win and will try to take back what has been taken away from it; That's nature, nothing personal.

2. Trying to lose 20 or more pounds, while trying not to eat the way you have been eating for the past 8,000, 10,000, 15,000 or more days, is a hard thing to do.

3. Trying to eat half of what you have been eating while others have a full plate and are eating the things that will not help you with your goals, is a very difficult thing. Temptations are all around us.

4. Trying to lose weight while managing a house, kids, and work is a very difficult thing to do.

5. Trying to lose weight while having some medical or mental issues, or while taking care of someone that has medical or mental issues, is a very difficult thing to do.

If you have one of the above items, you are entering a difficult journey! If you have more than two items, you are dead meat. ☹

It's your responsibility to take action if you want to lose weight; nobody else can do it for you!

It's very interesting how adults always want others to take control of themselves, when they can't self-control.

It's your responsibility to take action if you want to lose weight; nobody else!

You are the only one who can hold yourself accountable for your eating habits. Nobody else!

People are self-governing. You Govern what you eat, nobody else.

In life, Actions speaks louder than words.

Nobody can work harder than you in reaching your own goals!

MAKE A DECISION TO CHANGE.

COMMIT!

If you eat Avocado and Avocado oil today...

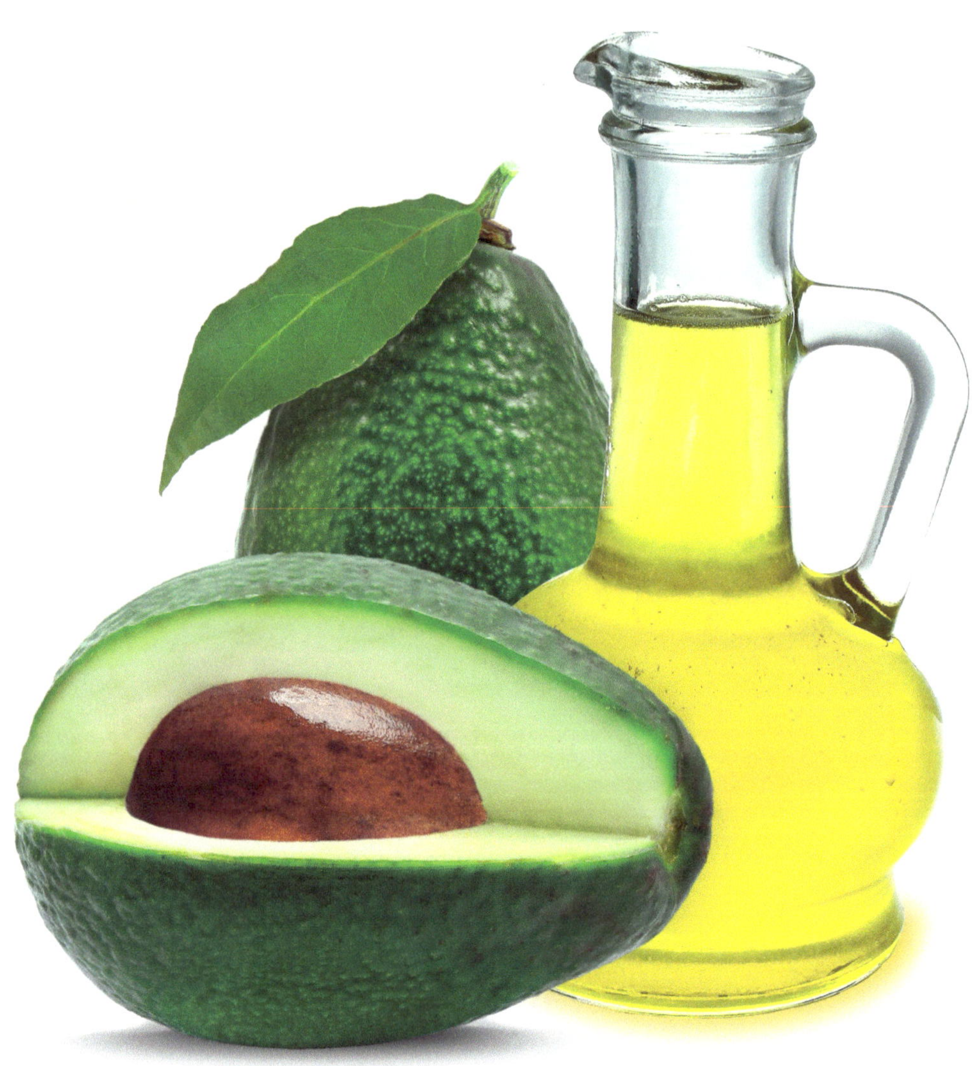

Then tomorrow you could be closer to...

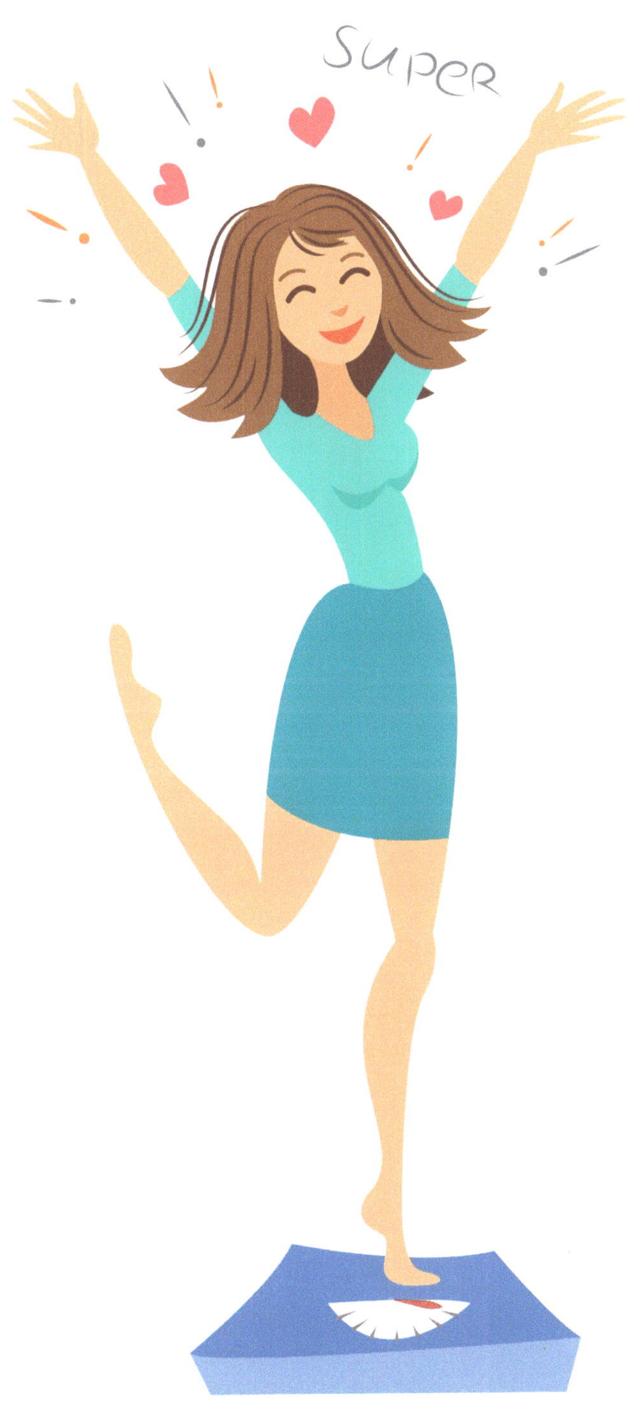

If you eat some cheese today...

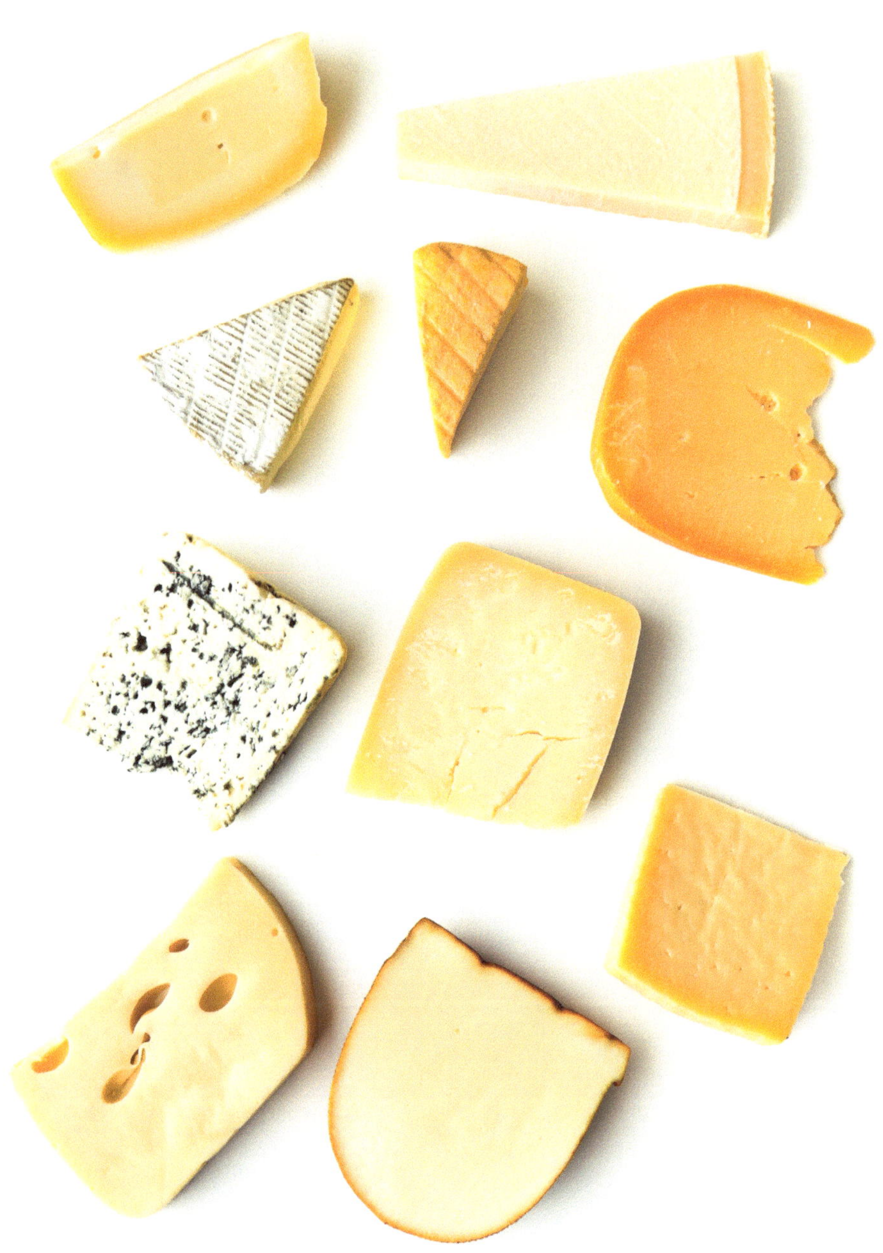

Then tomorrow you could be closer to...

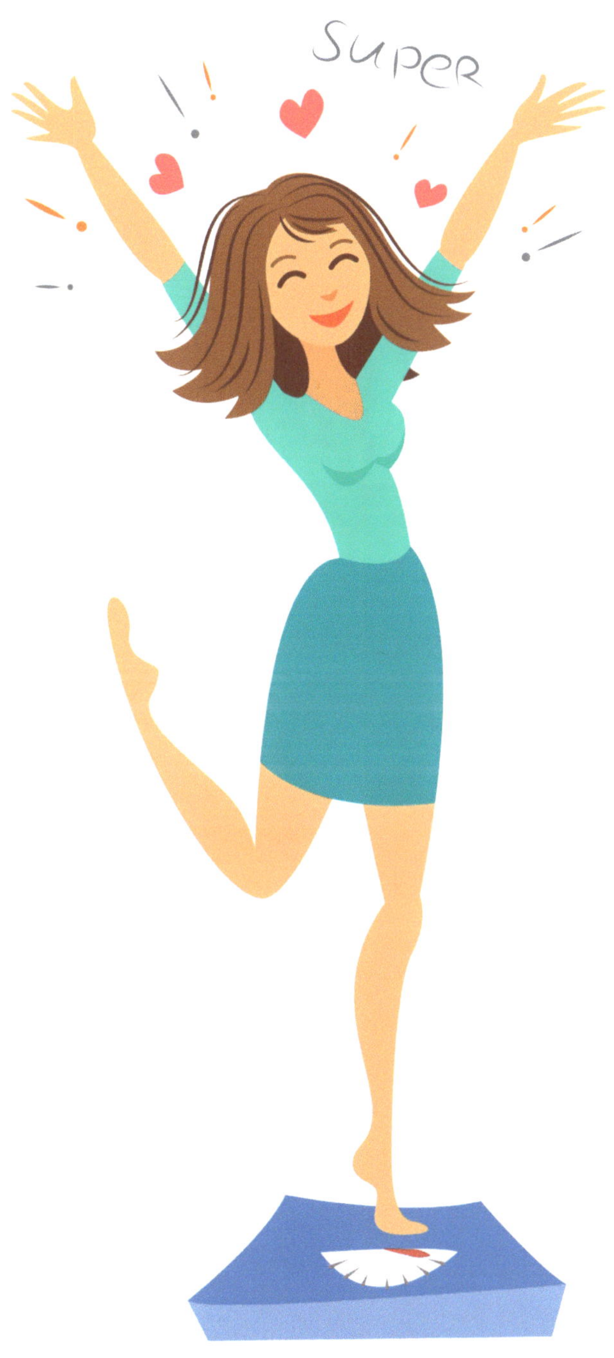

Be aware of the sugar in your drinks!
SUGAR, YOUR #1 ENEMY!

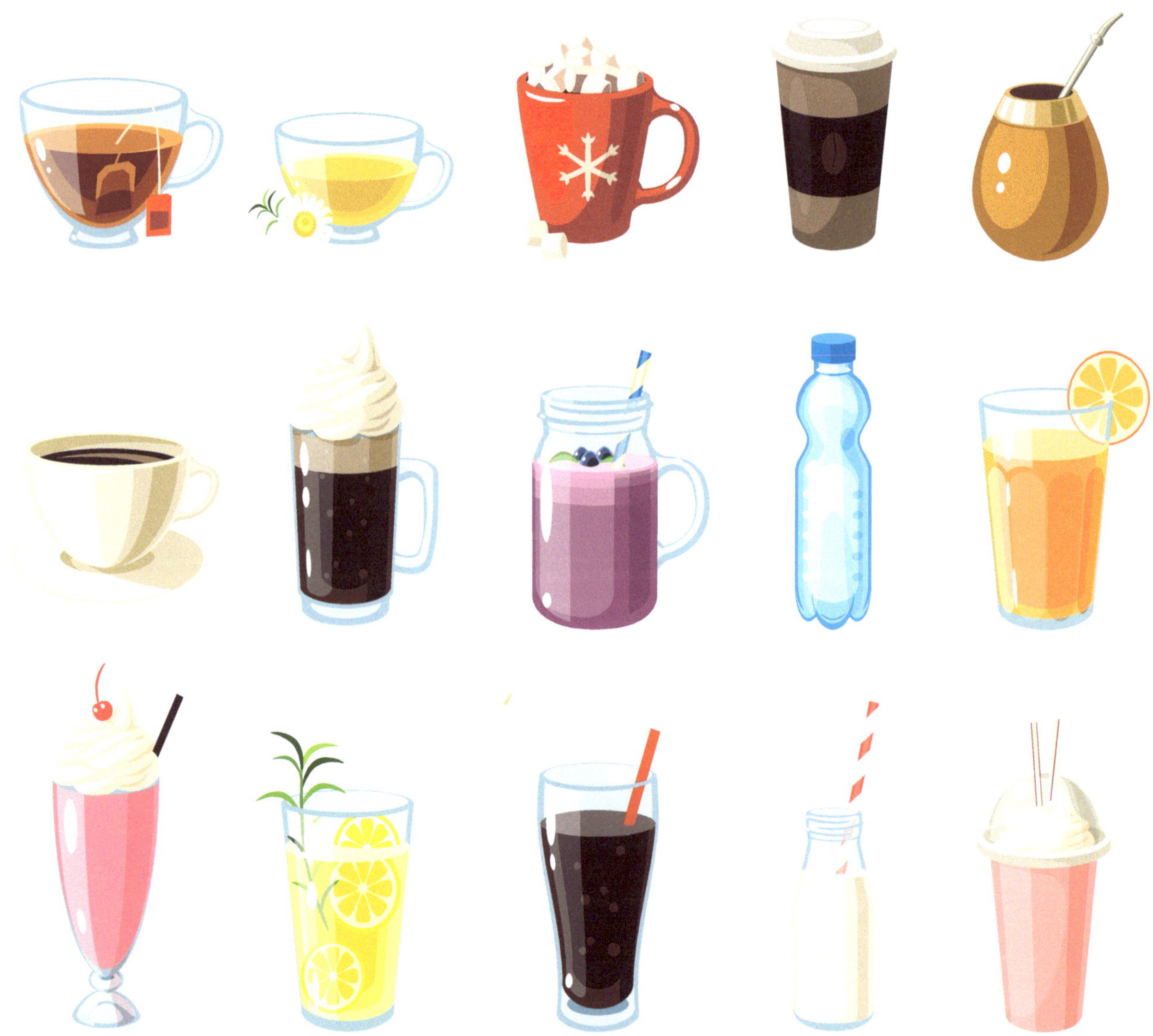

Use only Stevia, or Splenda as a second choice.

Your choice!

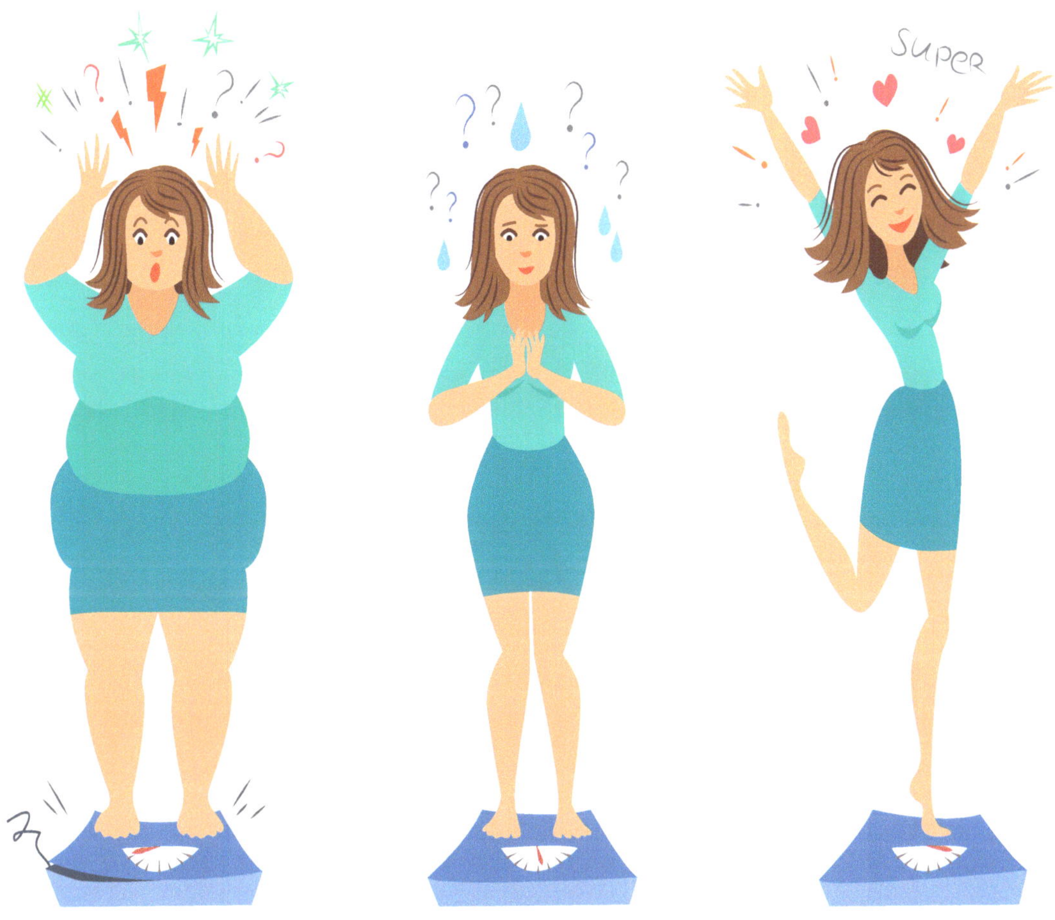

Sugar   Splenda   Stevia

If you eat eggs today...

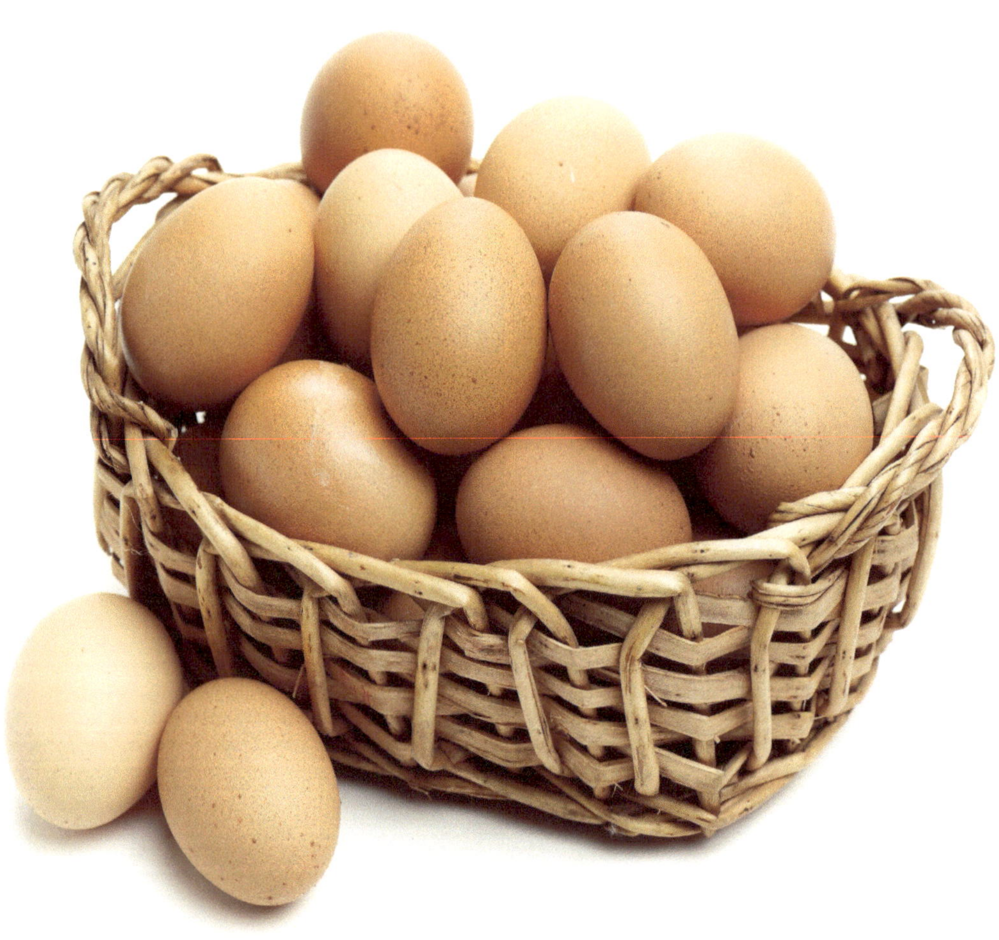

Then tomorrow you could be closer to...

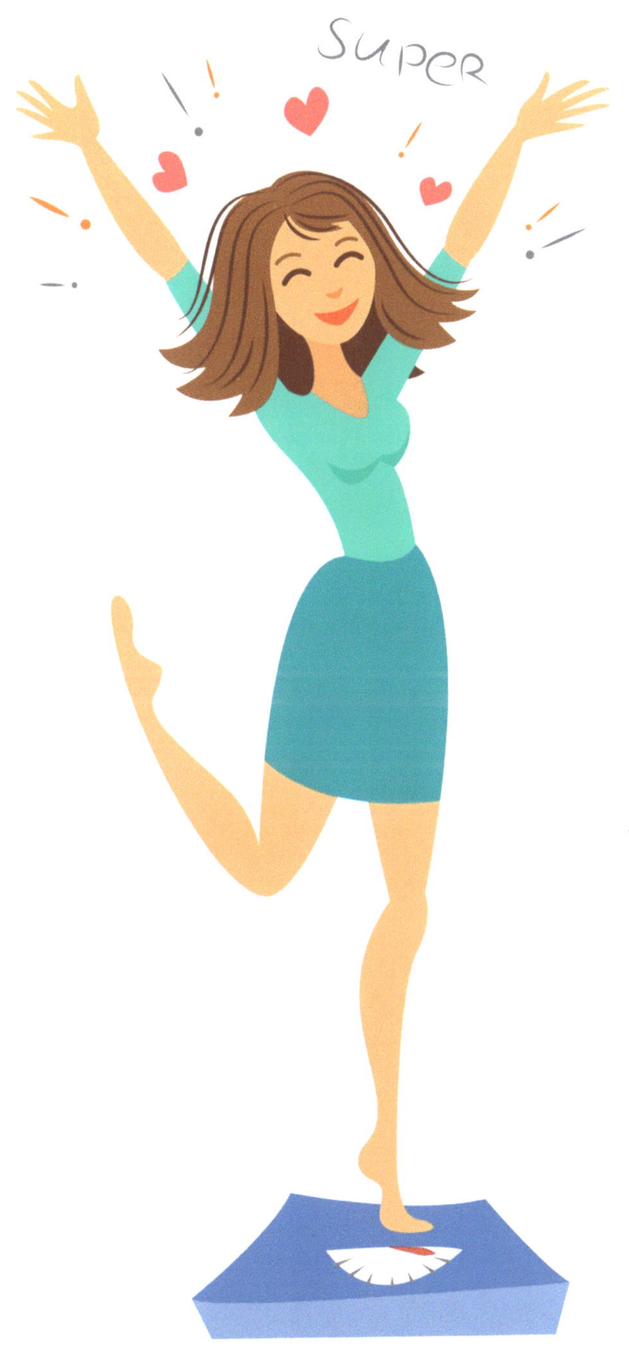

Take cold showers. Or, take hot showers and change the temperature to cold in the last minute of your daily morning shower!

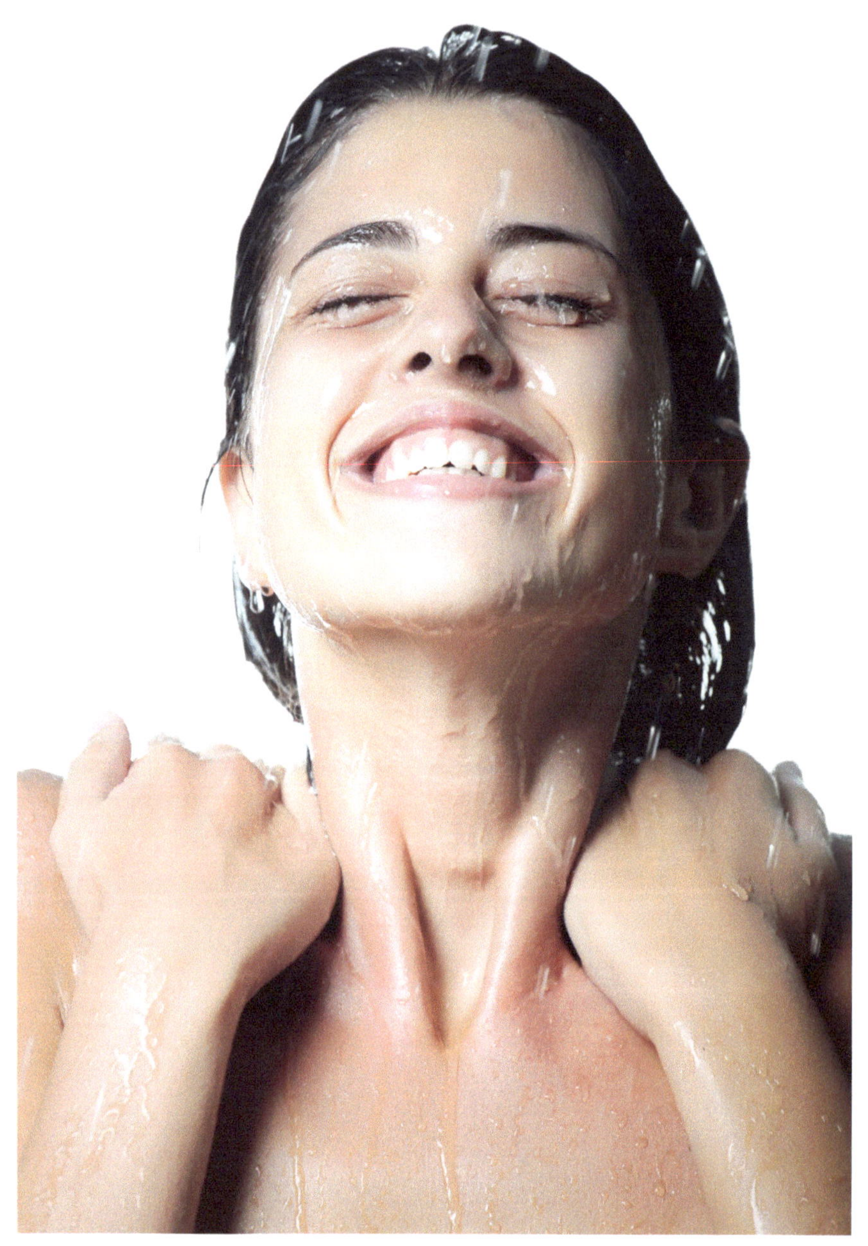

Energy, Will Power, Alert!

Then today you could be closer to...

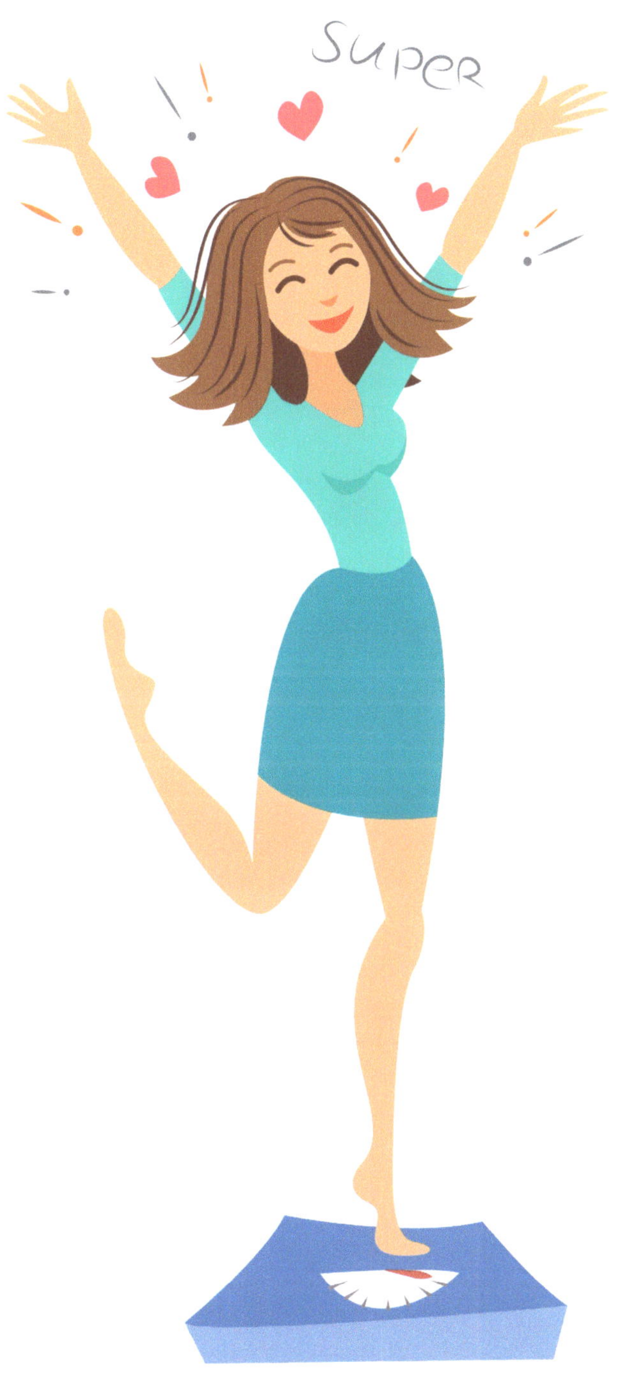

Replace RICE with QUINOA!

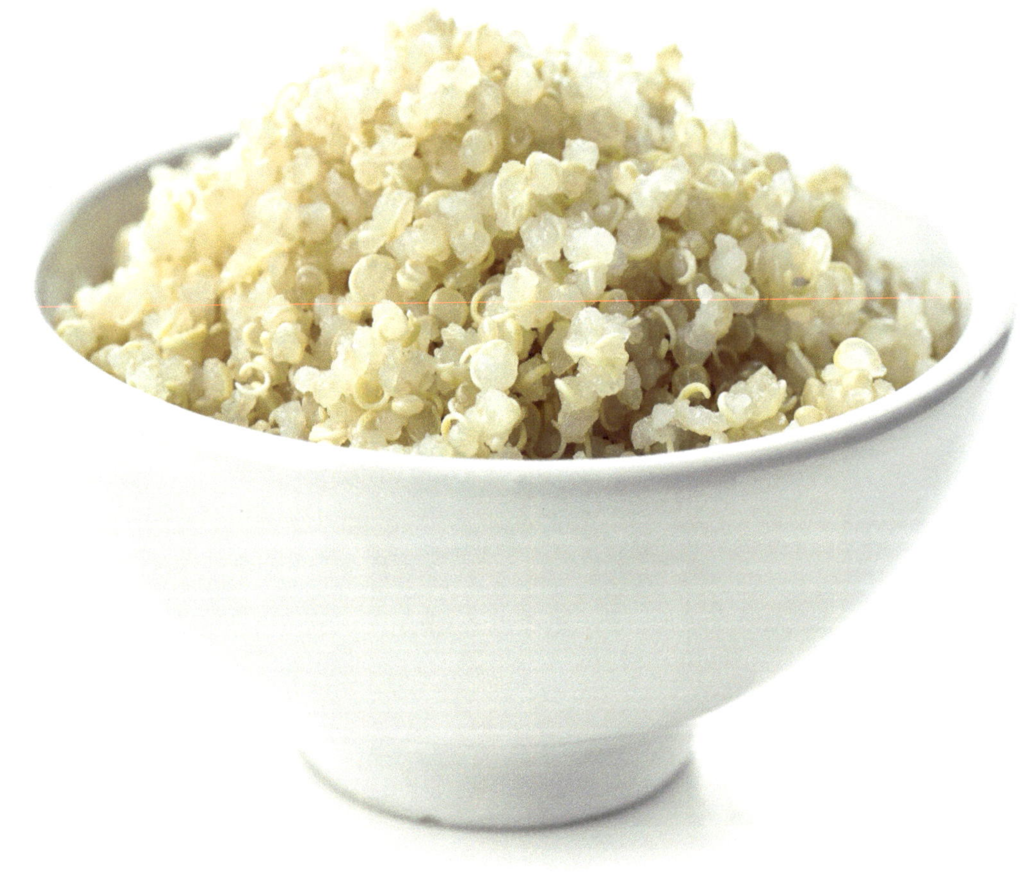

Your choice!

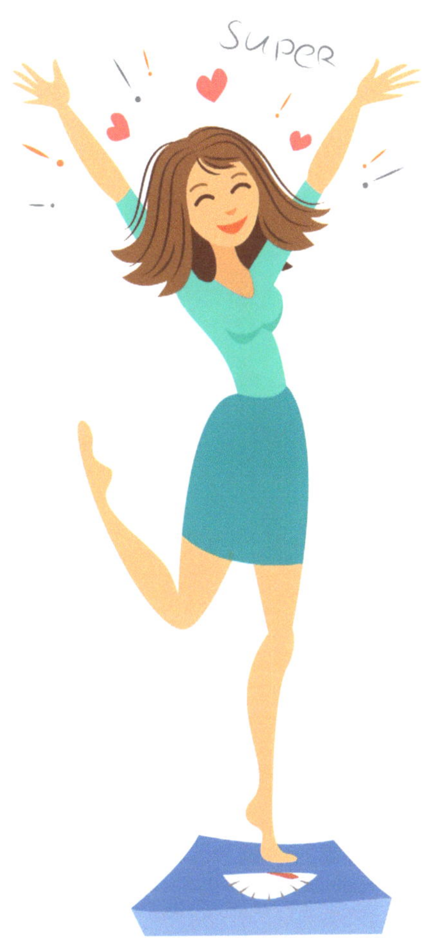

Quinoa

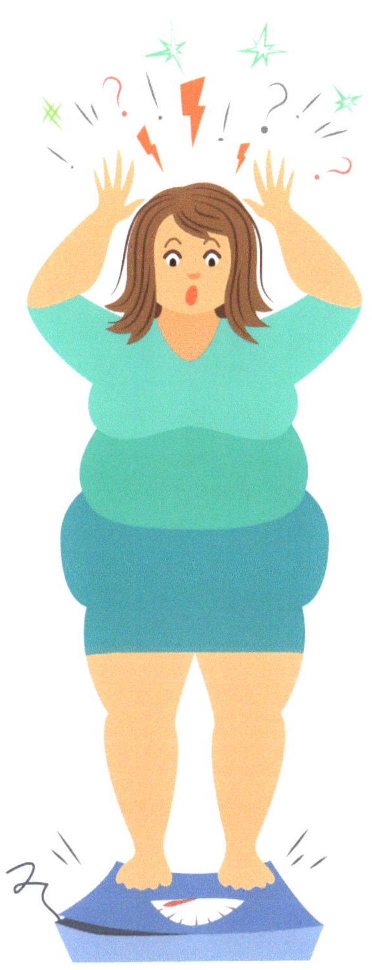

Rice

If you eat some nuts and seeds today...

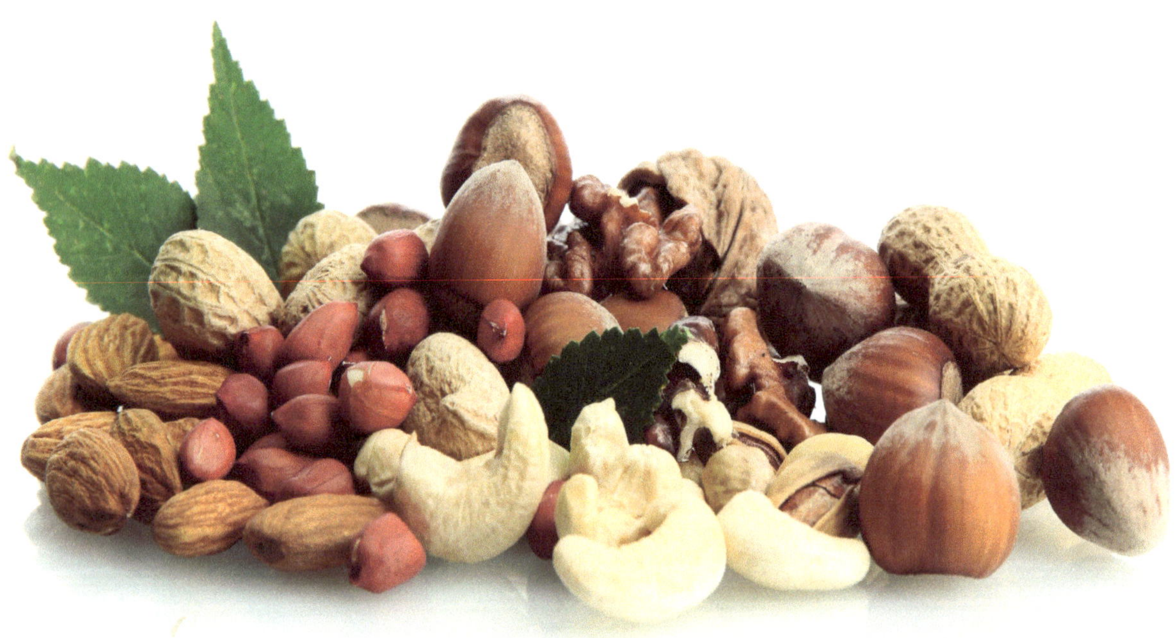

Then tomorrow you could be closer to...

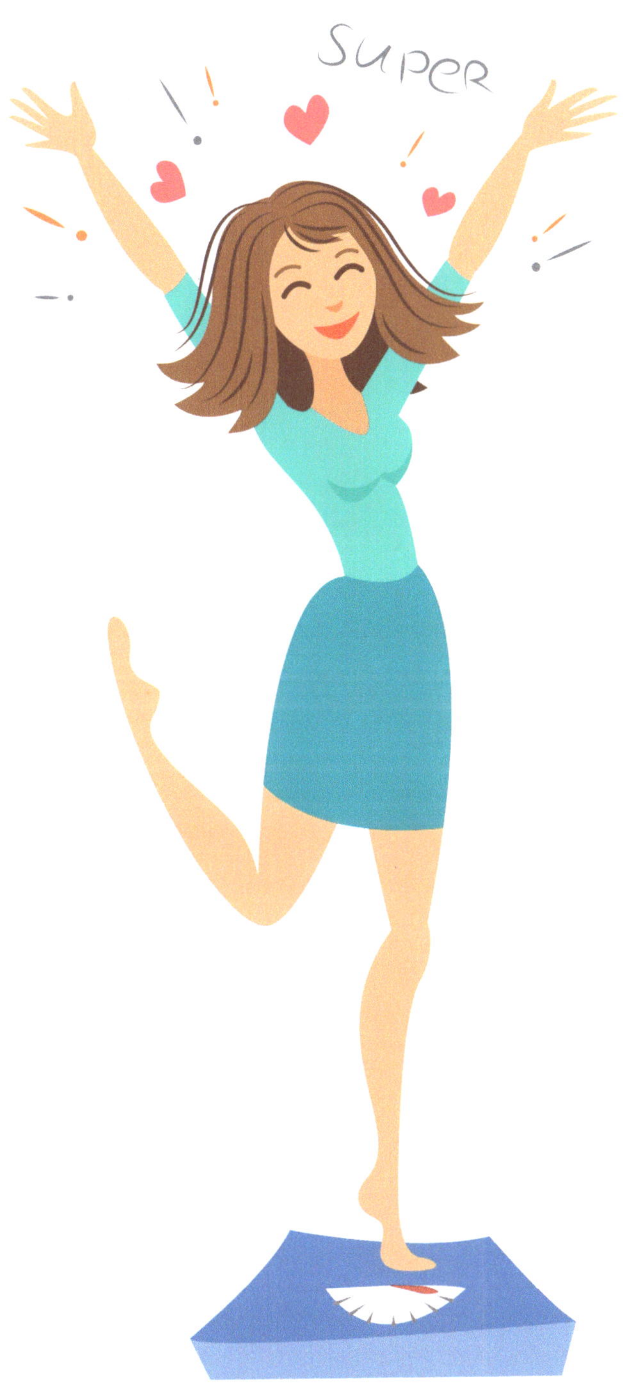

Don't Forget!

Less than 30g carbs = losing lots of weight

Between 30-50g carbs = losing little weight

Between 50-70g carbs = losing No weight

Over 70g carbs = gaining proportional to the intake of carbs.

This is the golden table for managing weight!

It's not easy, but it is your CHOICE!

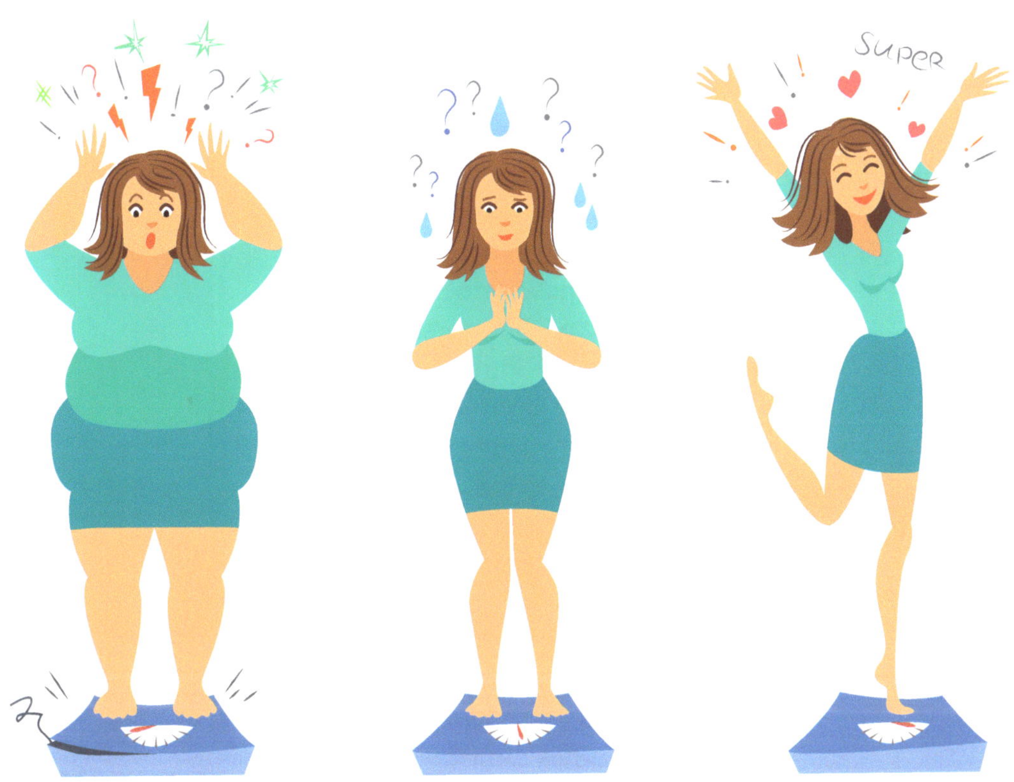

What is YOURS Today ?